# Troubles of Children and Adolescents

*of related interest*

**How and Why Children Hate**
A Study of Conscious and Unconscious Sources
*Edited by Ved Varma*
ISBN 1 85302 116 4 hb
ISBN 1 85302 185 7 pb

**How and Why Children Fail**
*Edited by Ved Varma*
ISBN 1 85302 108 3 hb
ISBN 1 85302 186 5 pb

**Violence in Children and Adolescents**
*Edited by Ved Varma*
ISBN 1 85302 344 2

**Group Work with Children and Adolescents**
A Handbook
*Edited by Kedar Nath Dwivedi*
ISBN 1 85302 157 1

**Meeting the Needs of Ethnic Minority Children**
*Edited by Kedar Nath Dwivedi and Ved P. Varma*
ISBN 1 85302 294 2

**How We Feel**
An Insight into the Emotional World of Teenagers
*Edited by Jacki Gordon and Gillian Grant*
ISBN 1 85302 439 2

**Something to Draw On**
Activities and Interventions using an Art Therapy Approach
*Carol Ross*
ISBN 1 85302 363 9

# Troubles of Children and Adolescents

*Edited by Ved Varma*

*Foreword by Valerie Sinason*

Jessica Kingsley Publishers
London and Bristol, Pennsylvania

The right of the contributors to be identified as authors of this work has been asserted by them in accordance with the Copyright, Designs and Patents Act 1988.

First published in the United Kingdom in 1997 by
Jessica Kingsley Publishers Ltd
116 Pentonville Road
London N1 9JB, England
and
1900 Frost Road, Suite 101
Bristol, PA 19007, U S A

**Library of Congress Cataloging in Publication Data**
A CIP catalogue record for this book is available from the Library of Congress

**British Library Cataloguing in Publication Data**
A CIP catalogue record for this book is available from the British Library

ISBN 1 85302 323 X

Printed and Bound in Great Britain by
Athenæum Press, Gateshead, Tyne and Wear

# Contents

# Foreword

In the last twenty years Ved Varma has been personally responsible for a significant number of invaluable textbooks. In fact he has been a one-man National Health Service within the field of publishing.

An Educational Psychologist and now full-time editor, he has kept his finger on the pulse of the subjects that evoke most clinical concern.

In *Troubles of Children and Adolescents* we see a genuine commitment to the wide range of skills provided by the multi-disciplinary team. This book provides thoughtful authors from a variety of disciplines (who also bring in research from other areas) so that psychology, psychoanalytic psychotherapy, behaviour therapy, family therapy, sociology, attachment theory, psychiatry, biology and ethology are all represented.

Experienced clinicans and authors like K. Eia Asen, Helen Barrett, David Jones, Francis Dale, David Fontana, Margaret Wright, Howard Roberts, Robert Povey, Tim Emms and Maurice Chazan together create a house style that eschews jargon and is clear to understand.

The authors know how to address key problems honestly and succinctly and with respect for clients and their families. The themes covered are troubles of relationships, anger, jealousy, withdrawal, aggressiveness, sexuality, adolescence, depression, learning problems, discipline and young offenders.

Whilst each chapter can be read on its own as a significant contribution to the theme it is devoted to, the book also reads as a very rich whole. Findng the similarities and differences between different theoretical approaches and techniques within the same profession, let alone between different professions, creates a greater understanding of the skills and resources available to children, adolescents and their families.

*Valerie Sinason*

# Introduction

Child psychiatrists, psychologists, psychotherapists, teachers and social workers deal with many children and adolescents with troubles. Those dealt with in this book are children and adolescents with troubles of relationships, anger, jealously, withdrawal, aggressiveness, sexuality, depression, learning and discipline, among others.

Susan Isaacs (1948) wrote that similar troubles crop up every year with each new family of children. Many of these troubles with young children are transient and normal, however trying to the parents they may be. They pass away with sensible handling and with further development of the children. Worried young parents seldom realise this. It is a great help to them to learn how frequent and typical such happenings are in the developing child. The mere lessening of anxiety in the parents through the knowledge that the early years of childhood are bound to have such storms and crises will do much to ease the difficulties of parents, and hence of the child.

But today the situation is much more complicated than in 1948. Hence troubled children and adolescents should be referred to experts as soon as possible. I also recommend this valuable and helpful book to professionals concerned with troubled children and adolescents in any way.

*Ved P. Varma*

## Bibliography

Isaacs, S. (1948) *Troubles of Children and Parents.* London: Methuen.
Freud, A. (1965) *Normality and Pathology in Childhood.* Harmondsworth: Penguin.

# CHAPTER 1

# Troubles of Relationships

*K. Eia Asen*

## Introduction

We are all born into families and, love it or hate it, the family continues to play a central role in most people's lives. During adolescence or adulthood even people who were permanently separated from their biological parents as babies become preoccupied with their birth families. It seems almost impossible to escape from the complex web of family ties, no matter how positive or negative the early relationships inside the family have been. It is in families that almost all of us form our first significant relationships. It is in families that children gain strength from closeness and it is here that they learn how at times their quest for independence can get suffocated.

From the moment they are born infants relate and are related to. In fact, it can be argued argued that it all begins *in utero* long before birth: many expectant parents treat their unborn as a person. This is made easier through the concrete evidence of ultrasound photographs of the foetus – to which the parents relate. Whatever the starting point, there can be little doubt that how children experience relationships inside their families crucially affects how they learn to relate to the world at large. Personal and relationship difficulties in adulthood can often be traced back to much earlier relationship troubles.

This chapter looks at how relationships are formed inside the family and how attachments develop. Common relationship troubles are described and ways of diagnosing and treating these are outlined. Since children mostly tend to experience relationship trouble inside the family, the major part of this chapter will focus on how family dynamics contribute and how the family can be used as a resource to overcome them. A brief section at the end describes how relationship trouble can be 'exported' to other settings – school, neighbourhood and peer relationships.

## The formation of relationships inside the family

Almost all of us learn about the making and breaking of relationships inside our families. Bowlby (1969) has shown how children's relationships with their parents are internalised as working models for relationships later in life. Securely attached children tend to explore their environment when they do not feel threatened. They are clearly affected by separation from their parents but immediately comforted when they are reunited with them. By contrast, infants who for one reason or another have not formed secure attachments to their parents show quite different responses. This can be shown by applying the Strange Situation Test (Ainsworth *et al.* 1978) which demonstrates how the quality of the attachments of infants to their parents affects their responses when separated from and subsequently reunited with them. 'Insecure ambivalent' infants tend to be distressed on separation and when reunited with their parents show prolonged anger and irritability. 'Insecure avoidant' infants, on the other hand, are not visibly affected by being separated and ignore their parent(s) on reunion. Research has shown that there are strong continuities from the quality of attachment in infancy to the handling of relationships in later childhood (Matas *et al.* 1978).

Much has been written about children's attachment to their parents and relatively little about the parents' attachment to their children. This is somewhat surprising, since attachment has to be a two-way process: the child's attachment to the parent is affected by the parent's attachment to the child – and who is to say what comes first?! Parents who are committed to their children will tend to produce securely attached children. Parents who are concerned with their child's welfare can provide safety, anticipate danger and take appropriate action. The result is that the child will feel contained. This containment is not merely an issue of physical safety, but has important emotional and cognitive aspects: the parents' capacity to reflect on the thoughts, feelings and wishes of the child is crucial for the healthy development of the parent–child relationship. It has been argued that 'good enough' parents are able to generate a variety of hypotheses and expectations regarding the state of mind of their children. At the same time they have the capacity to remain sensitive and responsive to their children's actual cues (Hill 1996) in the light of which some of these 'hypotheses' might need to be modified. It is bound to be a very intrusive and disqualifying experience for children to have parents who are convinced that they always know exactly what their child feels and thinks – no matter how much the child protests that he or she does not feel or think that way. Continued parental insistence on 'mind-reading' can seriously undermine the child's sense of self and result in self-doubt and confusion. Inevitably, relationship trouble develops with a variety of symptoms: for example, the child may increasingly withdraw and develop a very negativistic stance in relation to anything and everything the parent says. This is likely to be characterised by a seemingly endless string of automatic 'no's' to any parental suggestions. 'No' initially constitutes an act of self-preservation, but over time this will elicit negative responses from the parents and thus make the parent–child relationship increasingly troubled.

For children to develop healthily they need to grow up in a setting where the parents or carers are able to identify their offspring's central needs and concerns and take appropriate responsibility for their care. What makes parenting such a difficult task is finding a healthy balance between being sensitive to children's thoughts, feelings and need for experimentation, whilst at the same time being appropriately protective. The notion of the 'secure family base' (Byng-Hall 1995b) may be a helpful construct in this context: it provides a shared sense of security and belonging which gives every member, whatever his or her age, a 'good enough' sense of security to explore and grow. Each family develops its own unique attachment pattern and it is possible to study this in a more formal way by applying the Family Separation Test (Byng-Hall 1995a), a procedure designed for families with young children. The test is relatively easy to carry out and can be part of a family meeting convened by a clinician. Before the meeting the parents are asked if they are prepared to help with this test and they are given written instructions to leave the room at a given signal, leaving the children with the clinician. The parents are then asked to return to the consulting room after six minutes, entering the room together, standing side by side at the door for some five seconds before reacting naturally. The children are not informed about these instructions and therefore assume that it is their parents who are making the decision to leave the room. This test can give valuable information about difficulties in separating, caregiving between siblings during the separation from their parents, and shows which parent is the preferred attachment figure for each child on reunion. This test is one way of making a quick diagnosis of attachment and other relationship difficulties.

However, most clinicians may quite rightly feel reluctant to put children they see together with their parents through such a test and instead use other ways of 'diagnosing' relationship trouble. But what is 'relationship trouble'? It certainly is not an official psychiatric diagnosis and can therefore not be found in DSM and ICD manuals. It is a subjective 'diagnosis', made by family members or outsiders, denoting that there is something 'abnormal' going on between a child and other family members. Yet there is little agreement on what is normal and what is not. What is a normal relationship to some may well seem quite abnormal to others. People's own experiences of being parented tend to shape their expectations of how they themselves should parent. Parents who grew up in highly dysfunctional families may have much more tolerance of certain interactions, for example arguing, than those who developed in families where, difficult though this may be to believe, 'there was never a cross word'. On the other hand there may be those who think that such an absence of overt conflict is a sign of highly pathological family relationships! Moreover, what a grand-parent 'diagnoses' as relationship trouble, for example father shouting a lot at his sons, may seem utterly normal to the parent. Similarly, a father may be more worried than the mother about a problem and each could have very different views as to when that problem first started and how it manifests itself.

## Diagnosing relationship troubles

How then are typical relationship problems brought to the attention of a clinician? Generally they manifest themselves in two different ways: directly and indirectly. Sometimes parents are able to pin-point the problem, as they see it, directly: 'Jane can't get on with her sister and brother', 'Paul treats his mother like dirt', 'Annie has a very cold and distant relationship to her father' or 'Will is always very watchful when his step-father is around'. In these cases someone, usually a parent, gives a description of the child's perceived relationship problem. But relationship trouble can also present indirectly, namely with the focus on specific problems of a child such as bed-wetting, temper tantrums, stealing or very clinging behaviour. These are generally symptomatic of important underlying relationship issues.

There is plenty of potential for relationship trouble in each family: trouble between siblings, between the child and parent(s), between the parents and involving the child(ren), between the child and members of the extended family (above all grandparents) or a mixture of the above. Here are some examples:

- ○ a vicious jealousy between two brothers

- ○ a child who is continuously treated as a scapegoat

- ○ a child desperately getting involved in mending the parents' relationship

- ○ a young child 'parenting' the parents

- ○ a child very closely attached to the grandparents and utterly disrespectful of the parents.

It is possible that these or similar examples of relationship trouble may be directly reported by the parents when seeking help, but this is not always the case. On other occasions what may be obvious to any outsider goes quite unnoticed by the parents and other family members. It is the clinician's task to make sense of any direct or indirect evidence of underlying relationship problems. To do this a framework of thinking about relationships is needed. This means studying problems or symptoms within the contexts in which they occur, rather than simply focusing narrowly on the troubled child or troubled adult. It is not merely an individual whose problems have to be made sense of, but it is a whole relationship that comes under scrutiny. A suitable metaphor to describe this approach is that of a video camera which closely focuses on one object and then zooms back to a wide angle position. In this way the field of observation – and the site of intervention – is gradually widened. Such a 'zoom lens approach' is environmental, it creates new perspectives – not only for the clinician but also for the child and family. Once they get involved in this type of inquiry, child and family can look at themselves and each other from different viewpoints. It is a well-known fact that in relationships each person sees things from his or her very own perspective. The resulting failure to see anyone else's point of view often accounts for why things get stuck. If only those involved in a stalemate relationship could see their struggle from a bird's-eye perspective, things might come unstuck. It is often clinicians who can introduce the bird's-eye perspective. This is because outside observers are (hopefully) 'meta' to what goes on inside a family. Clinicians should be able to see the relationship trouble from multiple perspectives and in this way relationship problems are not seen as static or random events, but as events directly related to what goes on around the child.

What does this mean in practice? Clinicians who adopt a family relationships model can use ideas and techniques which challenge the very notion that problems are only located in just one person's genes, mind or brain. This can be done in a number of different ways, above all by asking questions which contextualise the child's relationship problems.

## Questioning relationship symptoms

The first step in any investigation is to ask questions. However, we need to distinguish between two kinds of questions. First there are those questions which clinicians ask themselves, the answers to which will help to understand the nature and dynamics of the relationship trouble. And second, there are those specific questions which clinicians will want to put directly to the family. These two types of questions are of course very much related, in that one informs the other. Yet, for conceptual reasons it is useful to distinguish between them, particularly since the first category, the 'hypothesising' type of questions, could not on the whole be put directly to children and their families. Let us turn first to this category and examine the following (Asen and Tomson 1992):

> *What* is the problem the child presents?
> function might the problem serve?
> is happening around the child when the problem occurs?

> *Why* is the problem present?
> is all this a problem *now*?
> *this* particular problem?

*When*  is the problem present?
   did it start?
   is the problem better?
   is the problem worse?

*Who*  is around when the problem happens?
   else has this or a similar problem?
   is most affected by the problem?
   is least affected by it?
   can make it better/worse?

*How*  does the problem affect the family?
   does the family affect the problem?

Answers to these questions will help clinicians generate ideas and hypotheses about the causes and contexts of relationship issues.

*What* problem the child presents may not necessarily be agreed upon by each member of the family (nor necessarily by the referrer). It can itself be diagnostic to listen to parents arguing with one another, disagreeing about what each regards as the child's actual problem(s). This allows the clinician to form hypotheses not only about the child, but about the parents' own relationship troubles. It is important to know what is a problem to who and it throws some light on the family dynamics if there are very different views held by different family members. For example, if mother believes that her son's relationship with his father is 'normal' whilst father believes it to be 'very troubled', then this tells us something about the family relationships. The 'complainant' is father who presumably wants a different relationship with his son. However, if mother does not regard this as an issue, where does this leave the son? In order to gain a better understanding of this the clinician will need to ask each family member very specific questions (for example, 'Mr X, how do you explain that your wife thinks your relationship with your son is "normal"?', 'Mrs X, in what way do you think your husband would like to improve his relationship with his son? Why is he worried about it?', 'John, do you know why your father thinks that your relationship with him is not good?' and so on). This form of questioning invites each family member to comment on relationships rather than requiring them to comment on personal feelings – they are examples of 'circular questions' (Selvini Palazzoli *et al.* 1980). This style of questioning can be described as 'interventive': the questions are not only designed to gather information, but above all make those questioned (family, child) think, hopefully setting a process into motion whereby they question themselves and their own belief systems.

The notion that problems can have a *function* may seem both strange and obvious at the same time. For example, in some families repeated acts of scapegoating a child may serve the function of preserving the domestic peace: the parents blame the child rather than each other. Implicit in this is the idea that if the child was no longer the scapegoat the parents might have a go at each other. In this way the scapegoating has a function as far as their own relationship is concerned. It should perhaps be noted at this point that this does not imply that a child deliberately 'decides' to become a scapegoat, or that the parents consciously gang up against their offspring in order to avoid tackling their own relationship issues. Instead it can be seen as a non-conscious interaction in which all are involved and which results in family members behaving in these particular ways.

*Why* problems occur is a crucial question for clinicians who want to uncover their primary cause. Looking for monocausal explanations, attractive though these may seem, rarely yields satisfactory results: most problems have more than one cause (genetic, temperamental, early experiences and traumas, social and cultural factors, current relationship issues and so on). Some or all of these can be simultaneously present and it may be very difficult to unpick with hindsight what came first. It can be helpful to focus on the present by modifying the why to: *why now* (rather than yesterday, last year or next month)? Clinicians want to find answers to the question: *why* is this relationship trouble *now* being brought to their attention? What is going on in the family now to bring relationship trouble to the attention of outsiders, including a request for help? There are many different specific questions which each family member can be asked (for example, 'If we had met two months ago, would you have said that the problems were different? What's happened since for you to come for help? What has made each of you decide that you should ask for help *now*?'

Another general question clinicians want to get some answers to relates to the issue of 'symptom choice': *why* is it that out of all the seemingly endless number of symptoms this particular one was 'chosen'? Clearly symptoms are rarely consciously chosen – they frequently represent a 'weakness' in the structure or system (a *locus minoris resistentiae*). A person with some (congenital) 'weakness' in the back will tend to develop back-pain when under psychological and/or physical stress. Similarly, a family system under stress may present with a symptom in one of its 'weak' parts: not infrequently the child. Viewed through the family lens the child's symptom – or the relationship problem that a child has with another family member – is a sign of system distress. When looking back over generations it is often striking how certain families tend to have specific patterns of somatisation ('in our family we all suffer from bowel problems', or 'headaches run in the family') or relationships ('in our family mothers do not seem to get on with their daughters' or 'I cannot think of a single man in our family who has ever been a good father'). Such deeply ingrained beliefs which seem to inform behaviours of family members have been called 'family scripts': unwritten recipes for everything from how to rear

children to the making and breaking of relationships. Each successiv
tion adapts the scripts handed down, hopefully taking on what se
and rejecting what makes no sense. Looking at family traditions, illnessc
patterns of conflict in families over time can often explain why certain problems
occur in a child or relationship.

Asking questions about *when* relationship trouble or other symptomatic
behaviours are present is important in that it provides further valuable information about context. Here general and specific questions overlap: the clinician
can ask direct questions about onset and course of the problem, enquire about
its fluctuation and elicit information about reinforcing or ameliorating factors.
Asking family members to identify times when relationship trouble seems to
be more marked helps them to identify those scenarios that are likely to make
things worse. It leads them to reflect on what action could be taken to avoid
unpleasant situations and, more positively, what could be done to have more
of those times when things seem to be better. In this way questions which seem
to be designed to elicit information become interventive: asking the family and
its members to reflect on alternative ways of conducting their relationships.

The various *who* questions have similar aims and can be put directly to the
different family members (for example, 'Who is worried about relationship
troubles? Who is most worried? Who is least or not at all worried?'). Asking
each person in turn will show how each family member may have different
perceptions about what (and sometimes even who) the problem is.

When considering *how* the problem affects the family and its individual
members, the most common answer one obtains is that it makes everyone
miserable and that it creates a bad atmosphere all round. It is only when
considering any possible 'positive' effects which the problem relationship may
have, that one starts thinking about the function of symptoms again. Many
symptoms regulate the distance between the various parties. For example, a
distant relationship between a mother and a daughter may suit father in that
his daughter is more likely to turn to him. He may consciously or unconsciously
fuel the conflict between his wife and daughter in order to protect his own
special relationship. It is possible for clinicians to get to this dynamic by
considering how the family and each member affect the problematic relationship: this gets away from the linear view of who is good and bad and introduces
the notion of 'circular' causality. Each family member may have quite different
views of who is to blame for what and how 'it' all started. For example, do
problems between parents 'produce' problems in their child? Or does a
problematic child produce strained family relationships? Clearly these questions
cannot be answered by an outside observer with a clear 'yes' or 'no'. Problems
develop in living contexts and even if one person appears to be more the cause
than the rest of the family, in the end everybody gets affected. Moreover, merely
by responding to one another all family members further affect each other. A

parent's response to his son's trouble will affect the son's responses, for better or worse, and other family members will react to what goes on between father and son – who in turn cannot help but respond to these responses…and so on.

Questioning relationship trouble is an important first step, both in terms of providing working hypotheses for clinicians as well as getting the different members of the family to question their own views. In this way the asking of questions becomes an intervention in its own right. Sometimes, however, responses to such questions can seem fairly abstract for children and their families, who will get tired of addressing hypothetical scenarios. After all, they have come with concrete problems and want them to be changed as quickly as possible. They cannot see the point of being asked all these questions – they want to change relationship trouble rather than have it endlessly questioned or analysed. It is in these situations that clinicians may want to make use of 'live' observations and concrete intervention techniques.

## Studying relationship trouble *in vivo*

Hearing about relationship trouble is one thing, observing it 'live' is another. There are times when clinicians cannot help but see troublesome relationships the moment they meet the family. Seeing the family sitting in the waiting room, with the parents and two children huddled together as a happy foursome and the oldest boy some ten feet away, hood over head and facing the wall – all this speaks volumes. The three-year-old toddler beating up his struggling mother who tries to get him out of the car is another example of relationship troubles being instantly visible – and audible. Many clinicians will use this as a starting point and work on what is there in the 'here and now', pointing out what they see and getting the family and its members to respond.

However, families often present themselves as united when first meeting a clinician in a new environment. It is then quite difficult to imagine how little Jenny, angel-like in the consulting room, could be the monster her parents make her out to be. Parents can be quite embarrassed as the child's immaculate behaviour seems to make them out to be liars. Yet, in such an event relationship troubles can be recreated and enacted in the 'here and now' during a family session: this allows both observation of what goes wrong as well as providing an opportunity for experimenting with new (re-)solutions. The clinician can invite the child and members of the family to demonstrate the 'trouble'. This technique is called 'enactment' (Minuchin 1974): parents and child are asked to re-enact the problematic behaviour. The clinician can elicit enactments by saying the following: 'Your child is now as good as gold. What would change that? What is it that you would have to say or do now for your child to show the sort of problems that have brought you here?' This directly encourages the parents to 'provoke' the child into problematic behaviour. Such 'instructions' seem to go against the grain, both of professionals as well as of parents. After all, clinicians are meant to improve matters rather than asking for trouble. However, once parents identify the 'switch' that produces dysfunctional behaviour, all hell can break loose. Parents are frequently quite unaware that they have the power to produce a crisis and that they have a part to play. Yet they have no trouble in identifying what they have to do to produce the problem behaviours: whether it is to ask them to sit down on a chair, to clear a toy away or to eat up their supper. Soon escalations happen, with the interactions reaching crisis point: here the clinician can not only observe the sequence of behaviours, but also help parents to look, on the hoof, for new (re-)solutions. In this way observation and therapeutic intervention become linked.

This approach shows how assessment and therapy overlap: observing how the various family members relate to one another gives an opportunity for intervention. Assessing their responses helps to predict the potential for change. An example is the first meeting with a family where both parents argue with one another, with their 5-year old daughter getting slowly drawn in. The parents' arguments are getting louder and their daughter becomes more and more demanding. The clinician predicts that any minute now the parents will stop arguing with one another, turn to their daughter and vent their irritation on her. At this point the clinician has a choice about what to do next: to observe the whole sequence and see whether the prediction turns out to be correct – or to intervene then and there. If the clinician chooses to do the latter, assessment turns potentially into therapy. Yet, at the same time the responses of the family and its individual members give the clinician the opportunity to assess to what extent there is a wish to see things differently and experiment with new ideas.

Here is a five-step framework for making use of *in vivo* observations, both for assessment and therapeutic purposes:

1. Observational statement
   (Clinician: 'I notice that you both raise your voices and that the louder you both talk, the more irritable your daughter becomes, so much so that you yourselves are getting annoyed with her')

2. Checking question
   ('Is that the way you want it?')

3. Clarifying inquiry
   ('How would you like it to be?')

4. Solution oriented question
   ('What would you have to say or do now to make it be the way you want it?')

5.  Generalising inquiry
    ('How could you ensure that what you've done here could happen
    between now and next time we meet?')

In this framework the clinician first highlights a specific interaction that may
be symptomatic of relationship problems. In the above example we hear about
a child that gets caught up ('triangulated') in a fight between her parents. There
are many other possible scenarios: a close relationship between a mother and
her son which leaves the second child out; a child who is continuously
disqualified by one parent and simultaneously praised by the other; two siblings
who fight violently in the presence of their onlooking parents – and so on. The
clinician deliberately 'punctuates' such a sequence by making the observational
statement (step 1), followed by the question: 'Is that the way you like it?' This
question is essential in that what the clinician identifies as 'trouble' may be
'normal' to the family and the family's reply may well be a whole-hearted 'yes'.
However, in practice this is a fairly rare occurrence in that most parents (and
children) have similar thresholds for what they regard as unpleasant behaviour
or a problematic interaction. The checking question (step 2) is important in that
it signals the clinician's respect for a family's potentially different definition of
what they regard as normal or pathological. It implies that the clinician does
not assume that families need to agree with his or her normative models of
family life and interaction.

When the parents or other family members reply with a 'no' then the
clinician can begin with the clarifying enquiry (step 3): 'How would you like
it to be?'. This respectful question invites the parents (and other family
members) to outline their own view(s) of what might constitute a better
interaction or way-of behaving with one another. Coming to some agreement
may not be easy for a family and the process of struggling to achieve it can
often be therapeutic. Once agreement has been reached the clinician can
proceed by asking a solution oriented question (step 4): all people involved are
asked to consider in practice what to do then and there. It is an action paragraph,
encouraging the family to work out something specific that can be implemented
right away. Whilst families do tend to feel pressured by this request, at the same
time there is also some relief that practical issues get tackled with practical
solutions. This can be highly therapeutic – as long as the solutions are not
prescribed by the clinician, but come from within the family. If there is some
change within the family session then the clinician might want to see how this
can be maintained afterwards and possibly generalised to the home setting (step
5): this can imply 'homework' for the family who plans how to make therapy
happen between sessions.

*In vivo* observations and interventions can be very effective and, as described
above, it is possible to recreate and 'enact' problematic interactions in the

consulting room. However, the most naturalistic interactions between children and their parents are of course in their natural environment – the home. Home based work may be time consuming, but quite a few families feel more understood if they can demonstrate where specific relationship trouble occurs. But families also go out and experience problems with their children in parks, on public transport or in a supermarket. Why not observe families in these settings and intervene in precisely those contexts where relationship trouble becomes public?! Studying relationship trouble in natural contexts 'live' makes it possible to understand how sequences arise. In a fairly unique multi-family project (Schuff and Asen 1996) parents (and children) are asked to identify typical pressure points of family life and these can be enacted in the community, whether it is on a busy street, on the underground, in the zoo, supermarket or pub.

## Relationship trouble outside the family

Children who have had the experience of a 'secure family base' tend to have the capacity to relate well to the outside world: what they have learned at home can usually be 'exported' to other settings – as long as the world outside is not too different! When children do experience serious long-term relationship troubles with their peers one needs to look more closely at how and where this happens. Is the child a 'loner'? Is the child unable to keep friends? Is the child always finding the 'wrong sort' of friends? What are the contexts in which relationship trouble is being experienced?

School is the most common place where such troubles manifest themselves. Obvious signs are bullying or being bullied, school refusal or disruptive behaviours in the classroom. Characteristically the school will blame the home and the parents in turn will blame the school for the problems. Children who bully may have 'learned' this behaviour at home. Or they may be bullied and intimidated at home so much so that they will want to take their own frustration out on some victims at school. But the school's responses to bullying will very much affect the child's behaviour. It is here that a joint approach, involving family and school, can help to improve matters (Dawson and McHugh 1994).

There are children whose self-esteem seems to be based on being the clown or having the reputation of being a 'toughie'. They generally feel very much undervalued and frequently underachieve academically. Gradually they develop a role and identity and they get noticed for it. Unfortunately much of this is based on negative attention and the teachers' and classmates' responses tend to reinforce troublesome behaviours. It is particularly children who have no friendships who carve out such identities for themselves and gain some dubious popularity. It is not surprising that such behaviours at school frequently reflect relationship trouble at home.

Parents can help their children to develop friendships. But for some parents the very thought of their children being more interested in the outside world than the home is quite unsettling. The 'parentified' child, looking after a sick or dependent parent, will find it very difficult to establish relationships with peers. He will be pseudomature and behind, preoccupied with his parent's welfare and sacrificing his own childhood.

## Conclusion

Troubles of children and adolescents, no matter where these manifest themselves, are more often than not connected with the main setting in which relationships are formed: the family. This is why clinicians need to consider the family as a major site for assessment and intervention. However, parents often feel blamed, particularly when asked to bring everyone for 'family therapy'. An alternative approach is to enlist the help of parents and other family members to help the child in trouble. In this way the family becomes involved as a resource rather than as a scapegoat. This allows relationship trouble to be tackled *in vivo*: in the family.

## References

Ainsworth, M., *et al.* (1978) *Patterns of Attachment.* Hillsdale, NJ: Erlbaum.

Asen, K.E. and Tomson, P. (1992) *Family Solutions in Family Practice.* Lancaster: Quay.

Bowlby, J. (1969) *Attachment and Loss: Attachment.* New York: Basic Books.

Byng-Hall, J. (1995a) 'Creating a family science base: some implications of attachment theory for family therapy.' *Family Process 34*, 1, 45–58.

Byng-Hall, J. (1995b) *Rewriting Family Scripts.* New York: Guilford Press.

Dawson, N. and McHugh, B. (1994) 'Parents and children: participants in change.' In E. Dowling and E. Osborne (eds) *The Family and the School*, (2nd edition). London: Routledge and Kegan Paul.

Hill, J. (1996) 'Parental psychiatric disorder and the attachment relationship.' In M. Goepfert, J. Webster and M.V. Seeman (eds) *Parental Psychiatric Disorder.* Cambridge: Cambridge University Press.

Matas, L., Arend, R. and Stroufe, L.A. (1978) 'Continuity of adaptation in the second year: the relationship between quality of attachment and later competence.' *Child Development 49*, 547–556.

Minuchin, S. (1974) *Families and Family Therapy.* Boston: Harvard University Press; London: Tavistock.

Selvini Palazzoli, M., *et al.* (1980) 'Hypothesizing, circularity, neutrality: three guidelines for the conductor of the session.' *Family Process 19*, 3–12.

Schuff, G.H. and Asen, K.E. (1996) 'The disturbed parent and the disturbed family.' In M. Goepfert, J. Webster and M.V. Seeman (eds) *Parental Psychiatric Disorder.* Cambridge: Cambridge University Press.

CHAPTER 2

# Troubles of Anger

*Helen Barrett and David Jones*

*Anger*
But we'll make it a rule to be friendly and clever,
Even if we are beat, we'll be pleasant as ever;
'Tis foolish and wicked to quarrel in play,
So if I get angry, please send me away.

*(Anon: Temple 1970, p.187)*

## What is anger? The problem of definition

Few individuals are unacquainted with anger. It is a common emotion which
occurs in various forms and to varying extents all through the lifespan and, in
English, we have particular ways of talking about it. As Tavris (1984) suggests,
the metaphors we use are often along the lines of a mechanical hydraulic model,
as though we were rather flimsy or unpredictable containers of some danger-
ously hot liquid. We talk of simmering, fuming or boiling with anger, getting
steaming or hopping mad or puffing up with rage and indignation. As we
become more angry, we spit with rage, foam at the mouth and our blood boils.
Anger surges up, floods out, erupts, spills out, boils or bubbles over, and flashes
from our eyes. We go red, purple or white, we seem about to burst. We react
by containing ourselves, bottling it up, keeping the cap on it, holding ourselves
back, in or together. Or we lose control, blow up, explode, blow a gasket, flip
our lids, hit the roof or fail to keep our hair on. Other metaphors also dissociate
anger from rational or healthy human beings. For example, we rage and roar
like bulls or lions, go spare, bonkers, potty or mad, have fits, throw wobblers,
lose our rags, or are completely speechless, apoplectic or convulsed with rage.

Yet, despite the apparent coherence of these metaphors, anger, like many
other commonly used terms, means such a wide range of different things to
different people that, when it comes to formulating a precise definition, there
is surprisingly little agreement. There is also a tendency to use the terms anger

and aggression interchangeably. This trend is perhaps particularly pronounced among psychoanalytic theorists who conceptualise aggression both as a reaction to frustration and as an instinct or drive. These theorists see the same negative drive state as giving rise to a wide range of negative affects and affective conditions, for example: 'Love, longing, jealousy, mortification, pain and mourning accompany sexual wishes, hatred, anger and rage the impulses of aggression' (Freud 1942, p.34). Many psychoanalytic theories of development are based on the premise that it is only the defensive mechanisms employed by the ego that keep destructive urges in check. In this view, the young infant, whose ego is still poorly developed, is likely frequently to be overwhelmed by the primitive emotions of anger and rage.

Among psychoanalysts, though, there is considerable divergence of opinion regarding the distinction between anger and aggression and their developmental trajectories. Winnicott, for example, described anger as a relatively late development: 'You will understand that these thousands of relative failures of normal life are not to be compared with gross failures of adaptation – these do not produce anger because the baby is not organized yet to be angry about something – anger implies keeping in mind the ideal which has been shattered' (Winnicott 1988, p.98). Tending to stay closer to its etymological derivation (literally, *stepping towards*), Winnicott saw aggression as being manifested early in development and being more like energetic self-assertion which is unmindful of others rather than intentionally negative towards them.

Clearly, anger and aggression are independent entities. Anger can be present without aggression just as aggression can be present without anger (or violence), even if this is not always the case. Also, although anger has been described as a 'basic emotion' (Darwin 1872) which can be identified readily in facial expressions (Ekman 1980) and in the crying of neonates (Wolff 1966), there is little consensus with regard to its status as a biologically-determined response (or set of responses). Kitayama and Markus (1994), for example, stress that the study of emotion has tended to reflect an ethnocentric bias. They argue that the ability to identify emotions across divergent cultures should be taken as evidence not for biological 'pre-wiring' but for the operation of varying psychological component processes within a commonality of social and cultural contexts.

## Cultural differences in the expression of anger

Wide differences have been found in parental practices relating to the socialization of emotion displays. In respect of anger, there is considerable cultural variation in the nature of anger-eliciting cues, in responses to those cues, in rules governing when anger may or may not be appropriate and in display rules.

Ellsworth (1994) proposes that in cultures where there is an emphasis on human agency and individual enterprise, anger may be more readily experienced and more dimensions of emotional appraisal may be operative. These dimensions include attention to changing conditions, the sense of certainty or uncertainty, perception of an obstacle, the sense of being in control, attribution of agency, awareness of impending praise or ridicule and judgement of the fitness of what has happened. For example, in Western industrialised cultures where autonomy and personal control are valued, it would seem that more dimensions of appraisal are used and negative appraisals are more readily made. In these cultures, there is a greater readiness to perceive disrespect and to demonstrate this perception with a display of anger, though the nature of this display will vary according to the rules in operation (Harris 1989). In some Latin cultures, for example, anger may not be recognised unless it is accompanied by loud and flamboyant displays and, amongst males in some Middle Eastern Arab cultures, failure to express anger is considered dishonorable (Tavris 1984).

Beliefs about the usefulness of anger also vary. For example, in North American culture, it may be considered healthy to express anger in order to feel good, clean and clear of emotional traffic jams (Rubin 1970). By contrast, the Utku eskimos strongly condemn feelings of anger, tend not to attribute blame so readily, make fewer negative appraisals and rarely use the the dimension of agency: 'It is no wonder that the Eskimos, who expect anyone who has reason to control his or her anger, make exceptions for children under the age of four, idiots, the very sick – and the *kaplunas*, white people' (Tavris 1984, p.177).

Wierzbicka (1994) also points out that language reflects and reinforces these different cultural understandings. The Ifaluk indians, for example, have no word for anger, admonition being the closest approximation, and in Polish different ways of describing anger can indicate whether or not its expression is socially acceptable.

It is also well established that the socialisation of anger displays in boys and girls varies according to socially constructed gender role expectations (e.g. Whiting and Edwards 1992). In many Western cultures, young boys, though more harshly reprimanded than girls for non-compliance, are often also subtly encouraged to display less inhibited, fiercer behaviour. Older girls who commit antisocial or delinquent acts, conversely, have been found to receive harsher punishments. It has also been found that already by age four, girls exhibit greater expressive control than boys in response to disappointment, although these differences have not been found to be accompanied by sex differences in the understanding of display rule usage (Tervogt and Olthof 1989). In an early study, though, Goodenough (1931) found greater variability in angry behaviour among boys and girls than between them.

## Towards a working definition of anger

Acknowledging the lack of agreement on a definition of anger, Smedslund (1993) outlines six possible approaches to a solution:

1. abandon psychological concepts entirely on the grounds that they do not describe anything that exists as a tangible entity

2. abandon the exercise of definition since everyone knows what anger is

3. accept that no one definition will suffice because the nature of anger is constantly being re-constructed

4. rely upon operational definitions alone (though the validity of these is threatened by their dependence upon non-operational definitions)

5. take the view that the construct of anger is a *fuzzy* concept, that is, made up of separate instances of anger which have little in common with each other but which bear some resemblance to an imaginary prototype

6. formulate a definition of anger based upon both classical definitions and more primitive concepts and axioms.

He dismisses the first three options as evasions rather than serious confrontations with the problem of definition. The fourth and fifth options he sees as rather more pragmatic but still not capable of yielding a satisfactory working definition of anger. He therefore opts for the sixth approach and, fashioning his theory of anger closely on accounts of aggression, proposes a definition of anger as 'a feeling involving a belief that a person one cares for has, intentionally or through neglect, been treated without respect and a want to have that respect re-established' (Smedslund 1993, p.30). He suggests that the person one cares for may often be oneself while being angry with things will arise only if things are endowed with anthropomorphic qualities (we only become angry when our cars break down if we construe the car as intentionally refusing to go, deliberately thwarting our aims and not respecting our needs).

In a preliminary exploratory study based upon a small sample of 24 respondents, Smedslund compared this *disrespect-anger* account with two alternatives: an *instrumental frustration-anger* account (analogous to the traditional frustration-aggression hypothesis) in which anger is viewed as a occurring only as a reaction to frustration of active attempts to achieve goals and a *general frustration-anger* account in which anger is viewed as arising from frustration of both active and passive goal expectations (such as wanting to be treated kindly). He presented scenarios describing different situations (specific to each of the three accounts of anger) in which anger may or may not be expected to arise and asked respondents to judge which situations would give rise to anger.

Ninety-six per cent of judgements appeared consistent with the *disrespect-anger* account, 72 per cent with a *general frustration-anger* account but only 24 per cent with the *instrumental frustration-anger* account.

A similar study by Harter and Whitesell (1989) investigating accounts of the causes of anger in three to eleven year-old children (divided into three age groups, 3–6, 6–8 and 9–11) lends tentative support to Smedslund's disrepect-anger account. Ninety-seven per cent of responses fell into two primary categories: 62 per cent were categorised as *physical or psychological pain* (e.g. being hit, having your feelings hurt) or 35 per cent as *things not working out as expected* (not getting something wanted or something unpleasant happening). Age of child was not associated with category of response. Harter and Whitesell suggested that violations of the self and unfairness were implicit in many accounts although their study did not explicitly measure this aspect.

Smedslund's *disrespect-anger* account is of interest in that it offers an alternative to the more traditional frustration-related explanations of the occurrence of anger. It is nevertheless problematic in some respects, for example, with regard to anger with oneself and with regard to anger in infancy.

In respect of anger with oneself, it is difficult to see how this could arise out of failure to treat oneself with due respect as this explanation suggests that the person who considers respect not due and the person who feels that insufficient respect has been paid (by the self to the self) must be one and the same. This objection may be countered if one thinks in terms of multiple selves, or of a self which is reprehensible at one time but not at another, or perhaps of a self within which different parts are in conflict. While these are uneasy solutions, they preserve the viability of Smedslund's definition.

A second difficulty arises in relation to anger in infancy and the feasibility of attributing infantile anger to infants' appraisal of respect for themselves or someone they care about. This definition appears to demand a sophisticated degree of social understanding which many theories of infancy would preclude, for example, seeing oneself from another person's perspective or even seeing other people as separate from the self. Again, this objection may be countered if one is prepared to accept that judgements about being respected need not depend upon conscious verbally-mediated processes. In this case, even very young infants might be sensitive to violations of their expectations with regard to level or quality of attention from significant others. Whether these violations would give rise to anger as opposed to other negative emotions, though, seems debatable.

A closer look at the nature and incidence of anger in infancy may help to throw light on these questions.

## The nature of anger in infancy

Belief that anger exists even in the earliest stages of infancy has been expressed by mothers (e.g. Pannabecker *et al.* 1980) and corroborated by research workers (e.g. Goodenough 1931; Emde, Gaensbauer and Harmon 1976; Sroufe 1977, 1979) and, as mentioned earlier, by psychoanalytic theorists. In a now classic small scale longitudinal study of the incidence and nature of anger during the first years of life, Goodenough (1931) described a gradual increase in incidence over the first two years of life with an apparent peak during the second year and a rapid fall-off after this.

Early manifestations of anger (or rage) can include crying, flushed and angry facial expressions, and increased motoric activity. Anger responses become more clearly differentiated by around the third month of life and are more frequent during the second half of the first year. From about the first year onwards, more co-ordinated behaviours such as foot stamping, kicking and throwing objects are in evidence. Restlessness, irritability, temper tantrums and sleeplessness are fairly frequent among children around 21 months of age and infants at this age display both anger and distress in reaction to pain. Izard and Malatesta (1987) suggest that anger may be more adaptive as a defence in mobile toddlers since it frees up more energy. It has also been suggested that children at this age are highly motivated to master both themselves and their environment. Angry responses at this age therefore contain an element of self-exploration or testing and may reflect a determined attempt to establish the conditions for self-respect rather than only to protect it.

By about two years, as language is added to the repertoire, responses become increasingly directed towards the source of the anger and defiant verbal expressions, biting, pushing and hitting are more common.

Although most workers have agreed that the earlier manifestations of anger or rage are far less differentiated or targeted than later expressions, there has been less agreement about how the earlier less well-coordinated behaviours relate to later emotional displays (Malatesta 1985). Sroufe (1979), for example, has argued that neonatal behaviour reflects primitive responses to extreme distress while true anger is more appropriately identified in the third quarter of the first year when some degree of intentionality is evident and anger becomes directed at and indicative of an awareness of a frustrating other. Other workers have been more willing to identify angry affective tone in neonates although these workers also acknowledge the reflexive nature of early responses (Emde, Gaensbauer and Harmon 1976). This dispute has important implications both for an understanding of the role of emotion in behaviour throughout the lifespan and for an appreciation of the nature of this role.

## The role of emotions in the behavioural repertoire

Until recently, with some notable exceptions, it has been usual to consider emotions either as epiphenomena or as predominantly irrational and disruptive intrusions upon cognitive processing. This view characterised the behaviourist school of psychology and was largely responsible for the relative neglect of the study of emotions during the twentieth century. More recently, however, it has become more usual to view emotions as organisational constructs whose main function is to organise responses.

This organisation has been seen as particularly important in relation to intrapersonal and interpersonal relationships and is thought to function on at least three levels in behavioural terms. First, on a conceptual level, emotions are thought to provide coherent summaries of complex interactions which help in the interpretation of events and behaviour. Second, at a process level, emotions regulate both intrapsychic and interpersonal responses in social interactions. In this way, they serve to facilitate and mediate adaptive coping (when to heed cues, when to seek help, when to keep one's distance, when to seek to remedy asymmetric power relations, etc.). Third, at a social level, through language, emotions act as signifiers. Since they arise specifically in relation to the history, current state and goals of each individual, emotions provide opportunities for the social sharing of experiences and in this way facilitate and mediate social cohesion (Frijda and Mesquita 1994).

The chief function attributed by ethologists to anger appears to be social correction with the aim of ensuring conformity to standards, for example, an angry display by a dominant chimpanzee towards a challenge from a subordinate may restore and reinforce the existing power structure by inducing both fear and respect in the less dominant chimpanzee; alternatively, adding anger to a reprimand may act to emphasise the importance of obedience to the reprimand. However, since anger works directly on the offender and involves a demonstration of lack of respect towards either a specific or a general aspect of the offender's behaviour, there is a danger that, if it is not well received, it will evoke anger in the recipient. Indeed, it has been found that children who are prone to angry displays tend to be avoided or rejected by peers, or even subjected to retaliatory aggression (Denham 1986). Further, as the metaphors used to express it indicate, anger is not a comfortable emotion to experience, although there are large individual differences in sensitivity to this discomfort. There is therefore often a distinct element of risk involved in expressing anger. This means that, in order for anger displays to be effective, they need to be carefully regulated and sensitive to their social context.

Learning to recognise and control one's own angry feelings sufficiently to judge when it may be safe to give expression to them or when it may be better to hide or ignore them is therefore extremely important; equally valuable are the skills required for accurate identification and efficient coping with signs of anger in other people.

## Learning to recognise and control anger

Very young children are sensitive to and can distinguish between facial expressions though, by three or four years of age, they rarely use facial expressions alone as a cue to emotional state. After the age of two, they spontaneously comment on their own and other people's feelings and are aware of the possibility that other people may not feel the same as they do. As early as three-and-a-half, children can identify accurately situations which may produce anger although identification of situations eliciting more complex emotions such as guilt and shame does not come until about two years later. By five or six, children begin to be able to appreciate that other people's emotions can be hidden (Harris 1989) although they may have learnt to hide their own feelings long before this (Buck 1984). The capacity to acknowledge mixed feelings develops more gradually and depends upon the strength, nature and target of feelings. Not until around age ten do children acknowledge that feelings of opposite valence can be targeted towards the same person at the same time (Harter and Whitesell 1989).

There are, however, large individual differences in the development of these skills which can be affected by dispositional variables as well as interactive experience.

## Temperament

In the study of temperament, much attention has been paid to the importance of individual differences and whether these are measurably present and persistent throughout the lifespan (e.g. Kagan et al. 1984). Early work by Thomas, Chess and Birch (1968) indicated that some infants were noticeably more prone to fuss, more difficult to soothe, less able to self-soothe and more intense in their reactions, that is, noticeably less able to regulate their own emotional state than others. This emotional self-regulation is thought to involve control of incoming emotional or otherwise arousing stimuli (attentional control) as well as responsiveness to internal cues relating to one's emotional state (Derryberry and Rothbart 1988).

Subsequent research has suggested links between infantile 'irritability', 'negative emotionality' and a range of adaptive behaviours, such as psychological difficulties, maladaptive coping, problem behaviour at school, poor quality parental relationships and resilience to stress (Lerner and Lerner 1986). It would appear, though, that the link between emotional arousability and behaviour problems is not a straightforward one since high arousability (dispositional level of reactivity, threshold and intensity of responses) in combination with high self regulation and good coping skills has also been found to be associated with social competence, including sociability, empathy and popularity. There is some indication that it is the combination of high arousability, low adaptiveness and high distractibility which may be linked with later problem behaviour.

There has been considerable debate about how or whether emotion interacts with, moderates or is moderated by temperament. The temperament construct of negative emotionality, in many temperament measures, relates to proneness to exhibit anger, fear and distress responses. Not surprisingly, this construct has been found to be highly associated with reactivity, arousability, irritability or being considered difficult to manage. However, since many temperament measures have not been independent of considerations such as caregiver behaviour, it is difficult to identify whether difficult or fussy infant behaviour leads to or arises from relatively unresponsive caregiver behaviour (Crockenberg 1986).

### Temperament and attachment

Some light has been shed on the relationship temperament and caregiver behaviours by some of the recent work on attachment using the Strange Situation procedure (Ainsworth and Wittig 1969). During this procedure one-year-olds are exposed to a novel play environment and separated twice from their carer, first in the company of a stranger, then alone. Infants' behaviour throughout the procedure and particularly towards carers on reunion is analysed to assess the attachment relationship between baby and carer. Of eight patterns originally identified (Ainsworth et al. 1978), four were described as secure (B1–B4), two as insecure avoidant (A1–A2) and two as insecure ambivalent (C1–C2). Secure attachment classification at one year has been associated during later childhood and adolescence with socially competent and adaptive behaviours, including popularity with peers, leadership qualities, self esteem, self-care skills, empathy, social skills, more satisfying interpersonal relationships and more effective problem-solving ability.

Temperament has not been found to be related to attachment security since infant fussiness, irritability or 'difficulty' is as common in securely attached as in insecurely attached babies. Further, although overt anger is most marked in ambivalently attached children, it is also thought that suppressed anger characterises the behaviour of avoidantly attached children. Despite the initial failure to find any systematic association between infant temperament and attachment pattern, Frodi and Thompson (1985) have suggested that children in the B3, B4, C1 and C2 attachment sub-groups are more emotionally expressive than children in other attachment sub-groups and that it may be the caregivers' management of children's emotionality which determines the nature of the attachment as well as the child's ability to learn how to control his/her emotions. In view of the fact that very few studies report data relating to attachment sub-group correlates, it is difficult to reach any firm conclusions on this issue at this stage.

Despite the difficulty of drawing specific conclusions about the relationship between emotionality, attachment patterns and later emotional adjustment, the attachment literature does give some indication that qualitatively different caregiver-child attachment patterns may be associated with children's ability to regulate their own emotional state and their skill in relating to emotional states in others. Similar findings emerge from research on the relationship between parental socialisation practices and children's ability to express negative emotions in socially acceptable ways.

### Parental socialisation practices

Children in families where negative emotions are frequently or intensely expressed are less likely to be able to identify emotions accurately either in others or in themselves (Dunn and Brown 1994) and it has been suggested that some interactive experiences are less likely to facilitate the development of effective anger management skills than others.

In a preliminary study, Eisenberg et al. (1992) looked at relationships between parents' responses to negative emotions in their children and the strategies the children adopted when confronted with anger-provoking, conflict situations with peers. More adaptive coping strategies (those which led to faster conflict resolution) and greater popularity appeared to be associated with parents' encouragement of expression of emotion as well as their acknowledgement and validation of children's emotional reactions. Less adaptive coping strategies (such as escaping or seeking adult assistance) tended to be associated with punitive parental responses while responses which minimised the children's emotional experiences were associated with more anger and less social competence.

In a later study, Eisenberg and Fabes (1994) used their Coping with Children's Negative Emotions Scale (CCNES) to identify six main strategies used by parents to cope with their children's expression of negative emotions: maternal distress, punitive responses, encouragement of emotion expression, emotion-focused coping, problem-focused coping and minimisation. Scores on the CCNES were correlated with observations of children's coping with negative emotion in social interactions at school as well as with parents' and teachers' assessments of children's temperament characteristics (emotional intensity, negative affect and attentional control). Observers coded seven coping strategies in children: verbal objection, venting, defending, physical retaliation, escape, re-engagement and seeking adults (the latter two were excluded from analyses due to low incidence).

Analyses indicated that supportive parenting, which acknowledged and enabled children to express their emotional responses and did not minimise or punish negative emotional experiences, was linked with constructive anger management in children; also mothers who perceived their children as able to self-regulate were more likely to adopt constructive strategies when confronted with their children's negative emotions. Positive correlations were also found between the maternal strategies of problem-focused coping, emotion-focused coping and encouragement of emotion expression. Minimisation and punitive reactions were negatively correlated with encouragement of expression of emotion, positively correlated with maternal distress as well as being associated with low attentional control and high negative affect in children. Further, maternal distress was found to be positively correlated with negative affect and emotional intensity in children.

While this data is suggestive in its demonstration of associations between mothers' ability to cope with children's negative emotions and children's ability to cope with their own negative emotions, the processes which might underlie such a fortuitous concatenation of maternal and child coping strategies are still not known. It has been proposed that positive adult role models may facilitate anger management in children as well as providing children with opportunities for talking about uncomfortable feelings without fear of ridicule or punishment. This might involve encouraging children to use increasingly precise and sophisticated emotion-relevant language (perhaps through stories and discussion of hypothetical situations as well as by discussion of real life events), helping them to feel more in control in situations where negative emotions are elicited, teaching them to notice when they are experiencing angry or hostile feelings and giving clear messages about which kinds of behaviour are likely to receive most social acceptance (Marion 1994).

Nevertheless, there is still much to be learnt about the most effective ways of managing anger and there is evidence to suggest that learning to use a range of coping strategies flexibly may be more important than perfecting the use of 'effective' strategies. Strategies, such as minimization or venting, may be maladaptive in one situation but adaptive in another. For example, it would appear that the strategies adopted by socially competent children are sensitive to power relations as well as to the nature of the anger-eliciting situation. Fabes and Eisenberg (1992) noted that even in pre-school children, strategies for coping with angry conflicts varied according to the degree to which the situation was perceived as controllable, the source of the anger (e.g. conflict over possessions, physical assault) and the differential status of the provocator (familiar or unfamiliar; adult or child).

Generally speaking, the more the situation is perceived as controllable, the more likely the child is to use strategies such as verbal objection and defending which maintain contact with and defuse the situation. In less controllable situations, children use strategies which may have negative repercussions for themselves or the other party, such as venting, seeking adult help or disengaging. Children who are popular, sociable and socially able will be far more likely to perceive themselves as in control than children who are prone to disruptive or anti-social behaviours, generally hostile or unpopular. Consequently, these children are less likely to feel the need to engage in displays of anger and more likely to experience positive emotion in social interaction (this, in turn, is associated with greater sophistication in emotion regulation).

### Anger management techniques

Training children who are impulsive and aggressive in the use of anger management techniques presents a challenge to therapists as well as to parents and teachers. Several intervention programmes have been developed based on cognitive behaviour therapy and rational emotive therapy. The initial stages of training typically involve helping the child to develop a greater awareness of when he or she is experiencing anger. Children can be helped to recognise some of the body cues associated with angry feelings. They may then be able to remove themselves from a potentially explosive confrontation. It is often possible to work out with the child a hierarchy of situations which give rise to anger responses. Unfortunately encouraging avoidance of conflict situations in real life is far from easy. For many children backing away seems like an admission of defeat or cowardice. With young children who exhibit frequent anger reactions in play it is sometimes helpful to focus on the more general area of development of social skills. They can be helped to experience the benefits of sharing, co-operation and other joint activities.

A somewhat different approach to helping children who have frequent angry outbursts is Michael White's technique of externalisation (White and Epson 1989). This approach is part of narrative therapy. Typically the child would be helped to find a word to label the behaviours which antagonise others. He (or she) would then be helped to distance him/herself from future repetitions of angry outbursts. The therapist might say 'What is it about anger which tricks you into getting yourself into trouble with your teachers?' The child may be encouraged to think and talk about the anger as a live entity with which he or she has a relationship. Attention is focused on the good times when explosions did not occur and the child is helped to build a picture of the self as someone who has control over emotions.

There is some similarity between the narrative therapy approach and psychodynamic approaches in that the latter too may aim to enable the child to construct a narrative in which anger is acknowledged as a response to serious internal conflicts. By recognising and respecting the child's anger and its role within the child's inner world, the therapist will seek to provide a relationship in which re-scripting can take place. In this way, the relationship between the therapist and the child may enable both recognition and containment of the child's more self-destructive tendencies: the therapist, like a receptive mother, will provide evidence that negative feelings can be inspected and tolerated and so enable the child to gain confidence in dealing with these difficult experiences. How the anger is woven into a self narrative, however, will depend upon the therapist's own schema or set of interpretations: Kleinian therapists, for example, usually operate with a unique set of assumptions and so make interpretations which can differ considerably from those of other psychodynamic therapists whose perspectives may be equally distinctive.

## Concluding comments

In their review and re-examination of meta-analytic data on outcome of therapy, Luborsky *et al.* (1993) re-affirmed, not completely unreservedly, that 'everyone has won and all must have prizes'. This 'Dodo Bird Effect' asserts that each therapeutic approach, whether psychodynamic, behavioural or person-centred, seems to have an equal chance of success and often contains common ingredients such as 'the support of the helping relationship with the therapist, the opportunity to express one's thoughts (sometimes called abreaction), and the opportunity to gain better self-understanding' (Luborsky *et al.* 1993, p.508).

Looking more broadly, though, at the extent of conflicts worldwide and the pervasiveness of violent images in the media, it is hard to feel equally optimistic about our ability as a species to manage negative feelings. Anger represents, particularly for those of us within Western cultures, a legitimate reaction to situations over which we feel we have little control. Avoidance of these situations is difficult if not impossible. As a result, anger remains a problem with which we all live, some more equably than others. It is hoped that in this chapter we may have thrown some light on ways in which children may cope and be helped to cope with their anger.

## References

Ainsworth, M.D.S., Blehar, M.C., Waters, E. and Wall, S. (1978) *Patterns of Attachment: A Psychoanalytical Study of the Strange Situation.* Hillsdale, NJ: Lawrence Erlbaum Associates.

Ainsworth, M.D.S. and Wittig, B.A. (1969) 'Attachment and exploratory behavior of one-year-olds in a strange situation.' In B.M. Foss (ed) *Determinants of Infant Behaviour, IV.* London: Methuen.

Buck, R. (1984) *The Communication of Emotion.* New York: Guilford Press.

Crockenberg, S. (1986) 'Are temperamental differences in babies associated with predictable differences in care-giving?' In J.V. Lerner and R.M. Lerner (1986) *New Directions for Child Development 31,* 53–73. San Fransisco and London: Jossey-Bass.

Darwin, C. (1872) *The Expression of Emotions in Man and Animals.* Chicago and London: University of Chicago Press.

Denham, S.A. (1986) 'Social cognition, prosocial behavior, and emotion in preschoolers: contextual validation.' *Child Development 57*, 194–201.

Derryberry, K. and Rothbart, M.K. (1988) 'Arousal, affect, and attention as components of temperament.' *Journal of Personality and Social Psychology 55*, 958–966.

Dunn, J. and Brown, J. (1994) 'Affect expression in the family, children's understanding of emotions, and their interaction with others.' *Merrill-Palmer Quarterly 40*, 1, 120–137.

Eisenberg, N. and Fabes, R.A. (1994) 'Mothers' reactions to children's negative emotions: relations to children's temperament and anger behavior.' *Merrill-Palmer Quarterly 40*, 1, 138–156.

Eisenberg, N., Fabes, R.A., Carlo, G. and Karbon, M. (1992) 'Emotional responsivity to others: behavioral correlates and socialization antecedents.' In N. Eisenberg and R.A. Fabes (eds) *Emotion and its Regulation in Early Development: New Directions for Child Development 55*, 57–73.

Ekman, P. (1980) *The Face of Man.* New York: Garland STPM Press.

Ellsworth, P.C. (1994) 'Sense, culture, and sensibility.' In Kitayama and Markus (1994) *Emotion and Culture: Empirical Studies of Mutual Influence.* Washington, DC: American Psychiatric Association.

Emde, R., Gaensbauer, T. and Harmon, R. (1976) 'Emotional expression in infancy: a biobehavioural study.' *Psychological Issues 10*, (Whole No. 37). New York: International Universities Press.

Fabes, R.A. and Eisenberg, N. (1992) 'Young children's coping with interpersonal anger.' *Child Development 63*, 116–128.

Freud, A. (1942) *The Ego and the Mechanisms of Defence.* London: Hogarth Press.

Frijda, N.H. and Mesquita, B. (1994) 'The social roles and functions of emotions.' In Kitayama and Markus (1994).

Frodi, A. and Thompson, R. (1985) 'Infants' affective responses in the Strange Situation: effects of prematurity and quality of attachment.' *Child Development 56*, 1280–1290.

Goodenough, F.L. (1931) *Anger in Young Children.* Minneapolis: University of Minnesota Press.

Harris, P.L. (1989) *Children and Emotion: The Development of Psychological Understanding.* Oxford: Blackwell.

Harter, S. and Whitesell, N.R. (1989) 'Developmental changes in children's understanding of single, multiple, and blended emotion concepts.' In C. Saarni and P. Harris (eds) *Children's Understanding of Emotion.* Cambridge: Cambridge University Press.

Izard, C.E. and Malatesta, C.Z. (1987) 'Perspectives on emotional development I: differential emotions theory of early emotional development.' In J.D. Osofsky, *Handbook of Infant Development,* 2nd ed. New York: Wiley.

Kagan, J., Reznick, J.S., Clarke, C., Snidman, N. and Garcia-Coll, C. (1984) 'Behavioural inhibition to the unfamiliar.' *Child Development 55*, 2212–2225.

Kitayama, S. and Markus, H.R. (1994) *Emotion and Culture: Empirical Studies of Mutual Influence.* Washington, DC: American Psychiatric Association.

Lerner, J.V. and Lerner, R.M. (1986) 'Temperament and social interaction in infants and children.' *New Directions for Child Development 31*, (Whole). San Francisco and London: Jossey-Bass.

Lewis, M. and Michalson, L. (1983) *Children's Emotions and Moods: Developmental Theory and Measurement.* New York and London: Plenum Press.

Luborksy, L., Diguer, L., Luborsky, E., Singer, B., Dickter, D. and Schmidt, K.A. (1993) 'The efficacy of dynamic psychotherapies: is it true that "Everyone has won and all must have prizes"?' In N.E. Miller, L. Luborsky, J.P. Barber and J.P. Docherty (eds) *Psychodynamic Treatment Research: A Handbook for Clinical Practice.* New York: Basic Books.

Malatesta, C. (1985) 'Developmental course of emotion expression in the human infant.' In G. Zivin (ed) *The Development of Expressive Behavior.* New York: Academic Press.

Marion, M. (1994) 'Encouraging the development of responsible anger management in young children.' *Early Child Development and Care 97*, 155–163.

Pannabecker, B.J., Emde, R.N., Johnson, W., Stenberg, C. and Davis, M. (1980) 'Maternal perceptions of infant emotions from birth to 18 months: a preliminary report.' Paper presented at the International Conference of Infant Studies, New Haven, Conn., (cited in M. Lewis and L. Michalson (1983)).

Rubin, T.I. (1970) *The Angry Book.* New York: Collier.

Smedslund, J. (1993) 'How shall the concept of anger be defined?' *Theory and Psychology 3*, 1, 5–33.

Sroufe, A. (1977) *Knowing and Enjoying your Baby.* Englewood Cliffs, NJ: Prentice Hall.

Sroufe, A. (1979) 'Socioemotional development.' In J. Osofsky (ed) *The Handbook of Infant Development.* New York: Wiley.

Stern, D. (1985) *The Interpersonal World of the Infant: A View from Psychoanalysis and Developmental Psychology.* New York: Basic Books.

Tavris, C. (1984) 'On the wisdom of counting to ten: personal and social dangers of anger expression.' In P. Shaver (ed) *Review of Personality and Social Psychology, Vol. 5: Emotions, Relationships and Health.* Beverly Hills, London and New Delhi: Sage.

Temple, N. (1970) *Seen and Not Heard: A Garland of Fancies for Victorian Children.* London: Hutchinson.

Tervogt, M.M. and Olthof, T. (1989) 'Awareness and self-regulation of emotion in young children.' In C. Saarni and P. Harris (eds) *Children's Understanding of Emotion.* Cambridge: Cambridge University Press.

Thomas, A., Chess, S. and Birch, H. (1968) *Temperament and Behavior Disorders in Children.* New York: New York University Press.

White, M. and Epson, D. (1989) *Narrative Means to Therapeutic Ends.* New York: Norton.

Whiting, B. and Edwards, C.P. (1992) *Children of Different Worlds: The Formation of Social Behaviour.* Cambridge, MA: Harvard University Press.

Wierzbicka, A. (1994) 'Emotion, language, and cultural scripts.' In Kitayama and Markus (1994).

Winnicott, D.W. (1988) 'Communication between infant and mother, and mother and infant, compared and contrasted.' In D. Winnicott, R. Shepherd and M. Davies (eds) *Babies and their Mothers.* London: Free Association Books.

Wolff, P.H. (1966) 'The causes, controls and organization of behavior in the neonate.' *Psychological Issues 5*, 1–105.

# CHAPTER 3

# Troubles of Jealousy

*Helen Barrett*

The problem of jealousy has been recognised throughout the history of humankind. The Bible, for example, tells how Cain's jealousy led him to murder his brother Abel, how a jealous Esau stole his brother Jacob's birthright and how Joseph's older brothers were angered by their father's favouring him. Indeed, in the Old Testament, Moses is given the Ten Commandments by a god who demands that he should be the only god to be worshipped 'for I the Lord thy God am a jealous God, visiting the iniquity of the fathers upon the children unto the third and fourth generation of them that hate me' (Deuteronomy 5:9; Exodus 20:5). It is in the image of this god that, according to the Old Testament, man was created: 'So God created man in his own image, in the image of God created he him; male and female created he them' (Genesis 1:27). These images of the pervasive power of jealousy have come to permeate literature within the Christian cultural tradition.

In Greek mythology too, with the story of Oedipus, Sigmund Freud found material to illustrate his theories concerning the universal importance of jealousy in the psychosexual development of young children. In this story, Oedipus' parents are warned by an oracle that their son will kill his father and marry his mother. In their anxiety to avert this end, they leave Oedipus on a mountain, to die. But a shepherd, Polybus, rescues the baby and he and his wife, Merope, bring him up as theirs. Learning of the prophecy and believing that his adoptive parents are his real ones, Oedipus leaves home in an effort to escape his fate. But he meets and kills Laïus, his father, and goes on to marry Jocasta, his mother, so fulfilling the prophecy.

According to Freud, this myth illustrates the playing out of an inevitable and universal desire on the part of the child for the exclusive attention and love of the opposite-sex parent. This desire brings the boy child into intense competition with his father. Because he dreads and objects to the loss of his mother's love, which he sees as rightfully his, the little boy is filled with hatred towards both his treacherous rival father and his traitorous mother. He projects his murderous intents into his father and becomes even more afraid of his father's revenge. Torn between his need for love and his jealousy, his intolerable conflict is eventually resolved by identification with his father, relinquishment of the demand for mother's exclusive attention and a subsequent diminution of respect for his mother. The triadic conflict is resolved and the child progresses to a more comfortable and socially-acceptable way of relating. Female children experience a less intense version of this Oedipal conflict (Freud 1933).

## What is jealousy?

Whether jealousy can be distinguished from envy has been disputed by theoreticians from many disciplines. Some have asserted that envy is associated with situations in which one desires attributes belonging to other people, for example, a smarter car, longer legs, more brains, etc. and that jealousy arises in situations where one senses that one's relationship with a loved person is threatened by that person's interest in someone else. In this view envy is seen as stemming from a two-person (dyadic) relationship whereas jealousy requires at least a three-person (triadic) one.

Other workers, though, have argued that since both jealousy and envy can give rise to similarly negative views of self and others and since they often occur together and are frequently used interchangeably in popular usage, there may be little heuristic value in distinguishing between them. Salovey and Rodin (1984), for example, have proposed that it may be more useful to speak of different types of jealousy which emerge from different situations: *social-comparison jealousy* which replaces envy and emerges in situations where one's status is challenged due to social comparisons on any dimension, *social-relations jealousy* where one's access to exclusivity in a relationship is challenged and *romantic social-relations jealousy* which replaces the term sexual jealousy. One difficulty with this taxonomy though is the implication that social-relations jealousy does not involve social comparisons. This clearly is not the case. In fact, it seems more viable to argue that it is in the nature of the social comparisons made that the crucial distinction may lie between jealousy and envy. Different situations may give rise to different kinds of negative social comparison and negative social comparisons made within triadic relationships may have greater potential for disturbing social relationships than those made within dyadic relationships. Two hypothetical cases can perhaps illustrate this.

## Envy: social comparison within a dyadic relationship

Simon, at three, is the only child of a young professional couple. Lively, robust and attractive, he has a warm, relaxed and friendly approach to other children. His best friend at nursery is Michael who is similarly well-endowed but slightly older than Simon. On his fourth birthday, Michael boasts that he is the oldest boy in the nursery. For once, Simon is not full of admiration for his friend. Instead, he is filled with envy. At Michael's party, he is grumpy about giving Michael the present he has helped to choose and reluctant to join in with games. 'When will I be four?' he asks his mother. 'Soon,' his mother assures him. The next day, at nursery, things are back to normal. Simon and Michael play together again.

Simon's envy made him temporarily dissatisfied with himself. It lowered his self-esteem and disturbed the usually good relationship between him and his friend. But it passed quickly because it was associated with very specific circumstances and involved comparison within a circumscribed area. For less well-endowed children, envy may be more generalised and its consequences may run deeper. But for Simon, in this instance, the discontent did not become generalised across other aspects of his social relationships and did not greatly affect his personality or general behaviour.

A rather different picture emerges from the next illustration.

## Jealousy: social comparison within a triadic relationship

Shortly after his fourth birthday, Simon's grandparents were tragically killed in a car accident leaving behind eleven-year-old Nessie, an adopted child, of whom Simon's parents were extremely fond. Arrangements were soon made for Nessie to move in with Simon's family. No effort was spared to help her to recover from her loss and to make her feel at home. Excited by the arrival of his young adoptive aunt, Simon revelled in the new situation and also shared his parents' interest in and enjoyment of Nessie.

Gradually though, as the toll of many rapid changes began to be felt, this situation changed. Nessie was not always willing to play with Simon on demand and Simon's exclusive relationship with his parents had clearly altered. Even so Simon often sought and readily accepted Nessie's attention. But, at night-times particularly, he would sometimes lie awake in bed listening to the hum of voices downstairs, knowing that while he was banished upstairs, Nessie was with his parents. Although he continued with his old routine of a night-time story followed by being tucked up by his mother, his discomfort and reluctance to go to bed grew.

Slowly, his behaviour changed. His general emotional state deteriorated and he became troubled by nightmares. During the day he often seemed distracted and unable to play in his usual spontaneous way. At times he looked tired and drawn, either in a world of his own or fractious, clingy and demanding. At nursery too there were reports that he was occasionally aggressive towards other children and less willing to play co-operatively than before.

In this vignette, Simon very much resembles two-and-a-half-year-old Gabrielle, better known as 'The Piggle' (Winnicott 1978). Her personality altered dramatically after the birth of her sister. For both Simon and the Piggle, the arrival of a third person upset the equilibrium of a relationship or set of relationships which was vital to their sense of self and self-efficacy. The third person constituted a threat which forced both children to review fundamentally their social identity.

Social comparisons made under these circumstances are not just along one or even several dimensions, in respect of specific attributes, but involve global considerations of one's worth as an individual. Each of these young children perceived the set of social relationships within which their social identity had been constructed to have altered so radically that they were no longer sure of their own value or meaning to other people. Their jealousy required that they re-think their self-concept in relation to the perceived attitudes of emotionally significant others. At a developmental stage when conscious, verbal articulation of abstract concepts is not accessible, they were alone in their struggle with the question of how to sustain a positive self-concept.

It is perhaps this alienating aspect of jealousy which has caused it to be considered so fundamental a problem in childhood. Young children are thought to be highly dependent upon attachment figures for both psychological and physical well-being. Since the jealous child perceives him or herself to be under-valued and deprived of the respect, love and admiration which has previously been regarded as his or hers by right, the resultant sense of exposure or betrayal inflicts a deep narcissistic wound. Unlike envy, therefore, jealousy presents a challenge to a child's sense of self in relation to important others. The child experiences this public challenge both as beyond personal control and as constituting a personal affront. Also, unless they are able to influence the child's perception of themselves, the emotionally significant others may well find a child who is jealous more difficult to cope with than a child who is more straightforwardly envious.

Particularly within psychoanalytic theory, where there is a heavy emphasis upon the formative nature of early emotional experience, situations evoking jealousy are seen as of fundamental importance because they represent an early separation/individuation experience between infants and caregivers. Such experiences are thought to influence children's internal representations and to set patterns for later social interactions. The child whose early experiences of envy and jealousy are not well contained or resolved is viewed as likely to become the adult who has difficulties in social relationships. Furthermore, although some workers in the psychoanalytic tradition have at times attempted to view sibling relationships from a more positive perspective (for example, Solnit 1983; Colonna and Newman 1983; Provence and Solnit 1983), many psychoanalytic theorists have proposed that sibling interactions, founded like other interactions on chaotic anti-social instincts, are essentially intensely hostile, threatening and underpinned by primitive and primordially destructive jealousy. How much evidence is there to support this view?

## Children's vulnerability to jealousy

As with many facets of children's emotional life, there has been much debate between workers in different disciplines about the nature of childhood jealousy. Since Freud's assertion that intensely hostile feelings between siblings are 'far more frequent in childhood than the unseeing eye of the adult observer can perceive' (Freud 1900, p.352), many psychoanalytic theorists and clinicians have continued to support the notion that envy and jealousy have a powerful impact on children's personality development in its early formative stages (for example, Adler 1921; Freud 1966; Isaacs 1948; Klein 1957; Levy 1934 1937; Oberndorf 1929; Stewart 1992; Winnicott 1978). In modern children's literature, too, the theme of sibling jealousy has often been given a higher profile than other aspects of sibling relationships (Begun 1979). Childcare manuals also have featured the theme, a typical statement being perhaps the following: 'jealousy is one of the facts of life and can't be completely prevented, so parents shouldn't expect to accomplish the impossible' (Spock 1945, pp.335–336). The belief that jealousy is a common childhood problem has therefore become widely accepted.

More recently though, over the past fifteen years or so, there has been a surge of interest in the study of sibling relationships among workers from more empirical traditions. Using a range of techniques including semi-structured interviews, questionnaires, surveys, observational studies, case studies and other qualitative methodologies, these workers have tended to take the view that jealousy is neither the distinguishing nor a ubiquitous feature of sibling relationships of young children. 'In the popular and clinical literature, the relationship between siblings is portrayed very much as one of rivalry and aggression, yet in home-based studies friendly, cooperative, and helping acts were frequently observed' (Dunn 1983, p.793). The general conclusion from these studies therefore is that prosocial behaviour occurs approximately two to three times more frequently than hostile or aggressive behaviour, that relationships between siblings often contain many positive features and that rivalry and aggression do not always imply the existence of jealousy (Dunn and Kendrick 1982; Dunn 1988; Dunn and McGuire 1992; Gottlieb and Mendelson 1990; Mendelson 1990).

Rivalry and aggression are seen as arising from many sources besides jealousy, for example, competition over possessions, disruption of treasured routines and intrusions of many kinds into what children perceive as their own personal space. But, given equitable conditions, processes have been documented which work towards mitigating the potential harm which might arise from rivalry. Schachter and Stone (1987, pp.72–73) argue that one of these processes involves differentiating oneself from the potential rival so that 'Left to their own devices, siblings are likely to find their way to normal deidentification, each with an equal, although different, share of life's delights'. In this view, then, rather than leading to serious difficulties, rivalry is seen more often to provide the motivation for resolving differences in the process enabling children to learn much-needed skills of negotiation, self-appraisal, co-operation and self-control.

Rather than considering jealousy to be an inevitable feature of children's emotional life, developmental psychologists have linked it with specific circumstances, for example, where children's personality is described as active and intense, where parents intervene inappropriately in sibling disputes (Schachter and Stone 1987) and where there is clear differential or preferential treatment shown towards one child, which may be particularly likely when siblings have an illness or a disability (Ferrari 1984; McHale and Gamble 1987; McKeever 1983). Also, it is emphasised that, even under these circumstances, individual responses vary tremendously and jealousy cannot confidently be said to be the distinguishing or predominant feature.

It is clear, then, that there are differences of opinion between workers adopting psychoanalytic and developmental psychology perspectives with regard to the role of jealousy in children's social and emotional development. Whilst it is beyond the scope of this chapter to resolve these differences or to judge between them, it does seem useful briefly to consider how they may have arisen.

## Ideological influences upon the understanding of jealousy in childhood

Three interacting levels of data-gathering can be seen to be potential sources of difference between workers adopting psychoanalytic and developmental psychology perspectives: identification, measurement and interpretation.

At the level of identification, no consistent definition of jealousy appears to have been agreed upon either in the psychoanalytic or in the developmental literature. Both groups of workers seem to have taken into account Darwin's categorisation of jealousy and envy as 'complex' as opposed to 'simple' emotions (Darwin 1872), that is, not shown directly through facial and bodily gestures (largely as in the higher mammals) but inferred from relationships between the individual and her/his social context. But there do appear to be differences in response to this problem. Within the developmental psychology tradition, there has been a tendency to formulate operational definitions. As a result, jealousy has tended to be seen as quite distinct from the negative emotional states associated with envy and rivalry and has been defined primarily in relation to situations in which it is thought to occur (Case *et al.*

1988; Fischer, Shaver and Carnochan 1989). Within the psychoanalytic literature, these distinctions are generally not made so clearly and the terms envy
and jealousy are often used as though self-evident, much in the way that they
are in popular usage.

With regard to measurement, psychoanalytic observations have been drawn
largely from individual clinical case studies while developmental psychologists
have used a range of research methods, some of which have involved larger-scale
longitudinal studies with more representative populations or experimental
settings. It is perhaps possible that over-reliance on overtly observable phenomena in the developmental literature may sometimes have been at the expense
of the understanding of children's intentions. This can work both ways:
negative interactions may mask positive intentions which misfire due to young
children's immature social skills but positive interactions, such as helping, may
mask an older child's need for domination (Newman 1994). Systematic research
in this area is still at a relatively early stage. It seems likely that the most accurate
picture will emerge from a mixture of qualitative and quantitative approaches.

With regard to interpretation, ideological differences are possibly most in
evidence. In theory, it is not clear which discipline, an empirically-based one
such as developmental psychology or a hermeneutic one such as the psychoanalytic tradition, would be more readily permeated by political influences. In
practice though, it seems possible that the physical composition of the work-
force within each discipline is likely to have an influence. An extremely élitist
group, such as the psychoanalytic establishment, may fare better in a society
which places a low value on its members' capacity for self-government. It will
be in the interests of highly élitist establishments to conceptualise individuals
as inherently anti-social or untrustworthy since fostering such beliefs is more
likely to maintain social order and thus reinforce the authority of the élite.

Despite these large differences concerning the nature of jealousy in childhood, there remain at least two important points upon which workers in both
traditions are agreed. First, both groups of workers agree that the birth of a
sibling is a stressful time in most families, that quarrels and fights are not
uncommon and that jealousy can be a serious problem which, for some
individuals, may endure throughout life. Second, they also agree that, because
of the way children cope with their jealous feelings, jealousy may be both hard
to detect and difficult for those closest to the child to help with.

## Jealousy across the life-span

Tesser (1980) proposes that, as there is an underlying need to maintain a
positive self-concept, spontaneous social comparisons should be associated
only with situations which are seen as self-relevant. It follows from this that
children will make particular types of social comparison according to their

maturational stage, experience and disposition; that is, individual differences in the nature and number of comparisons made will depend upon the child's self-concept which in turn will depend upon their developmental level and social experience. The child with aspirations to become a pianist will spontaneously compare herself to other piano-players and may be spurred on or cast down by her self-evaluation. The budding footballer will be prone to make comparisons and will feel vulnerable under quite different circumstances.

The concept of self is a huge issue which has puzzled thinkers across the ages and there is no intention here to engage in these debates. But it is well established that children's sense of self and their ability to reflect on their self-image changes as they mature (Higgins, Ruble and Hartup 1983; Stern 1985; Damon and Hart 1988). There is also evidence that the complexity of elements within the self-concept and the degree to which parts are differentiated and fixed alters fairly systematically throughout childhood, though these alterations vary considerably according to culture, social context and individual differences such as temperament or physical constitution.

It would appear that, as children become older and their self-concept becomes more distinctly defined, they make more spontaneous social comparisons along specific self-relevant dimensions. For older children, only negative comparisons made in domains of personal importance seem to be associated with strong negative affect. Further, comparisons which yield negative affect are generally with others who are perceived as of similar status to the older child. In other words, older children tend not to compare themselves with people who they perceive as very different from themselves, for example, people who are very much more advantaged physically or socially. By contrast, younger children make fewer spontaneous social comparisons and are more upset than older children by self–other comparisons in domains which do not appear to be of great personal importance (Bers and Rodin 1984).

Since the nature of negative social comparisons depends so heavily upon the elements which go to make up the child's self-concept, it seems possible that there will be distinct differences between the self-concepts of children who easily become jealous and those who do not. Research is still needed to address this issue but it may be the case that the self-concept of people highly prone to jealousy will be found to contain more global, static, absolute or superlative elements ('favourite', 'best', 'always', 'adored') as opposed to specific, transient or relative elements ('sometimes', 'good at sport', 'doing OK', 'getting there'). The ability to think in less absolute, less rigid and possibly more adaptive ways may be associated with cognitive and emotional level or attributional style.

No clear agreement appears to have been reached with regard to the first appearance of complex emotions such as envy and jealousy in childhood. As mentioned earlier, psychoanalytic theorists have suggested that envy is first ascertainable from birth. Others have proposed that social comparison processes cannot begin until a certain stage of cognitive maturity has been reached.

Young children often make illogical inferences which aggravate and perpetuate a vicious circle of negative social comparisons. Robey, Cohen and Epstein (1988) suggest that they believe that 'positive regard is a divisible substance of limited supply' (Robey et al. 1988, p.2): according to this naïve theory of affection a parent who loves someone else cannot love you too. While the jealous child believes, or perhaps only half-believes, that s/he no longer has access to exclusive love, s/he is not prepared to relinquish a claim on or a need for that love. Unable to see clearly from the other child's perspective and thinking in absolute rather than in more sophisticated relative terms, the young child may assume that the exclusive love is still available to the other child. On the basis of this misconception, the child may then experience his rejector as deeply hurtful, himself as deeply unlovable and the other child as a severe threat. Both the child's immature cognitive skills and the presence of erroneous premises mitigate against addressing the problem through rational discussion.

While some early work based on anecdotal accounts has suggested that the experience of jealousy is observable in children as young as three-and-a-half months (Gesell 1906), more systematic studies have tended to suggest that it is not reliably observable as a distinct emotion until somewhat later. Masciuch and Kienapple (1993) used an experimental design to measure the responses of 112 children (ranging in age from 4 months to 7 years) to mothers praising another child (either peer or infant). They concluded that, as predicted by the cognitive-developmental models of Fischer et al. (1989) and Case et al. (1988), it was rare for children under a year to manifest jealousy but that jealousy could be reliably and validly inferred in children older than one year. They described children aged between 1.1 and 2.3 years as being most prone to manifest jealous responses and also outlined developmental changes both in the strategies adopted by children to regain mother's attention and in the nature of the situation required to elicit jealous responses. Older children manifested jealousy only when they felt personally challenged. They also used more elaborate strategies to attract attention to themselves and away from the competitor.

With regard to children's understanding of jealousy in other people, a different time-scale has been proposed. This depends upon the child's having reached a fairly advanced stage of cognitive development at which there is an appreciation of other people's perspectives as well as a capacity to reflect upon one's own response to situations. Selman (1980) suggests that this understanding emerges in three stages. At level 0 (approximately 3–6 years) there is an emphasis on activities and concrete objects: people are not seen as jealous of other people but of the activities and objects they are in possession of. At level 1 (around 5–9 years) the focus is still predominantly on objects and activities but there is now a possibility of recognising that being excluded may be distressing. At level 2 (7–12 years) greater understanding of one's own and other people's feelings is available and the part played by being excluded from a relationship is now acknowledged. Work investigating this conceptualisation is relatively sparse and there seems to be evidence of quite considerable individual and cultural variation here.

## Cultural variations

On the subject of cultural variations in manifestation of and incidence of childhood jealousy, it is important to bear in mind that in many cultures, after infancy, very young children are not cared for by their natural mothers but, often, by an older child who may be a sibling: 'As a consequence, children tend to be highly peer-oriented, and uncomfortable in intensive one-to-one inter-action with adults' (Weisner 1982, p.309). This possibility seems to have received little attention within the developmental literature and almost none in the psychoanalytic literature.

Much more attention has been devoted to patterns of sibling relationships within Western-style nuclear families. In these families, particularly between brothers, it seems, co-operation is less likely and competition can be intense. But even in these families it would appear that siblings do act as attachment figures for each other; many, particularly sisters, have considerable under-standing of each other and may become increasingly able to act as confidants; further, in the main, rivalry appears to diminish across the life-span, although living together may re-activate earlier rivalrous relationships (Cicirelli 1982). These findings tend to re-affirm the view of sibling relationships as intense, capable of being both very good and very poor but, more often, being a mixture of good and bad. Over the life-span, physical and emotional distance may attenuate relationships but can also allow space for re-negotiation and repair.

## Coping with jealousy

It has been recognised that, once emotional expression comes under voluntary control, children soon learn to disguise their feelings (Blumberg and Izard 1991). Within psychoanalytic theory, it has also been suggested that the capacity to defend oneself against uncomfortable feelings and to minimise the risk of experiencing unmanageable anxiety begins as soon as the infant starts to experience itself in relation to its caregiver, that is, from conception. Much emphasis has been laid upon the role of primitive forms of envy. Particularly in relation to feeding, where the infant is unable to have omnipotent control over sources of gratification, it is thought that envy is in evidence. The resultant emotional state is so intense and intolerable that the infant develops a range of strategies to protect itself from experiencing its true state of helpless impotent dependency. In Klein's view, this primitive envy permeates all the infant's relationships and operates mainly at a pre-conscious level since, as the infant develops, increasingly sophisticated defensive mechanisms ensure that there is little need to consciously acknowledge or directly experience the raw emotion. Only in cases where normal defences have failed does the threat become more apparent.

The range of defensive tactics identified by workers within the object relations school is wide. For instance, infants may withdraw their emotional investment from the desired object, deny any need for it or denigrate it. Alternatively, they may salvage a sense of their own omnipotence by projecting negative feelings out into other people or things or by splitting the desired and unobtainable object (for example, the breast) into two separate imaginary entities (the good and the bad) with the good breast still being retained (introjected) as part of the infant and the bad breast being split off or projected into other objects. Further developments include evermore complicated mental acrobatics with the values attached to these imaginal entities being converted or dissipated or re-attached to other objects or activities. The underlying theme, though, is that there is a tendency for children to be defended against experiencing themselves as lacking in efficacy. They will not see themselves as consumed by the envy which fundamentally underpins their relationships with important others.

Something of these protective mechanisms is perhaps observable in Simon and the Piggle. Neither Simon nor Gabrielle appeared directly to experience him or herself as unlovable yet both seemed to suffer from a sense of loss of status or meaningfulness due to the newcomer's arrival. Unrequited desire, if not given up, almost inevitably becomes persecutory since it is not possible for it to be satisfied. Unlike Esau, Cain, and Joseph's brothers, Simon and the Piggle did not remove or attack their rivals. Instead, they protected themselves against the full impact of their aggression by converting the real threat into imaginary nightmare figures which nevertheless took a toll in terms of their ability to engage fully with everyday life.

In the Piggle's nightmares, she imagined a 'black mummy' and a 'babacar' both of which she appeared simultaneously to love and to hate, to need and to fear, that is, they represented both her positive and negative feelings about herself, the wanted object and herself in relationship with the object (they possibly also reflected some of her confusion about pregnancy and childbirth). These figures, frightening though they were, by externalising her own perception of damagedness and damagingness, served to keep at bay the tremendous threat to her sense of self. However, because they symbolised both desire and unmet desire, they were in danger of being able to maintain themselves at the expense of their creator. It therefore became very important for her to be able to use Winnicott, by whom she was given sixteen analytic sessions, to disown these creatures. Believing that Winnicott knew about and understood the black mummy and the babacar seemed to help the Piggle to come to terms with her fears.

This seems to raise the question of how necessary it may be for children suffering from jealousy to receive counselling. There seems little doubt that in most families the birth of a sibling is stressful, for parents and children alike (Dunn and Kendrick 1982; Vandell 1987). It is also true that many parents at times find their children's quarrelling and fighting extremely trying. But it is also the case that, where children are feeling excluded, the person best suited to help them is the one they feel excluded by. For this reason the most effective professional help will be that which enables this help to be given.

Where problems of jealousy are associated with other problems within the family, for example, marital disharmony, favouritism, the presence of a child with a disability or a terminal illness, the introduction of extra family support through a sympathetic befriending network can be very helpful. In addition, some families may benefit from more intensive family therapy work. Individual attention from trusted adults outside the family network may also be helpful and this may come from a variety of sources.

A major aim of support work with jealous children will be to enable them to see themselves as having their own social identity which is unique and valued in its own right. This may not always be easy to achieve as the children may need help in finding a sphere of activities which is both personally meaningful and not in competition with the children seen as their rivals. But, in most cases, help will come from within their immediate social network: from mother who continues, despite extra commitments, to respond positively to each child; from father who, after the birth of the new baby, assists more with caring for and developing the interests of the older child; from altered relationships with other siblings; from members of the extended family; from teachers, neighbours, friends or other people who are important to the child. Perhaps most importantly, help will come from within the child as he or she pursues his or her own inherent need for positive self-esteem.

## References

Adler, A. (1921) *Problems of Neurosis*. New York: Cosmopolitan Book Co., 1930 edition.

Begun, A. (1979) 'Sibling relationships as portrayed in young children's literature.' Unpublished manuscript, University of Michigan, Ann Arbor, Michigan.

Bers, S.A. and Rodin, J. (1984) 'Social-comparison jealousy: a developmental and motivational study.' *Journal of Personality and Social Psychology 47*, 4, 766–779.

Blumberg, S.H. and Izard, C.E. (1991) 'Patterns of emotion experiences as predictors of facial expressions of emotions.' *Merrill Palmer Research Quarterly 37* (1), *183–197.*

Case, R., Hayward, S., Lewis, M. and Hurst, P. (1988) 'Toward a Neo-Piagetian theory of cognitive and emotional development.' *Developmental Review 8*, 1–51.

Cicirelli, V.G. (1982) 'Sibling influence throughout the lifespan.' In M.E. Lamb and B. Sutton-Smith (eds) *Sibling Relationships: Their Nature and Significance Across the Life-Span.* Hillsdale, N.J.: Lawrence Erlbaum Associates.

Colonna, A.B. and Newman, L.M. (1983) 'The psychoanalytic literature on siblings.' *The Psychoanalytic Study of the Child 38,* 285–309.

Damon, W. and Hart, D. (1988) *Self-Understanding in Childhood and Adolescence.* Cambridge: Cambridge University Press.

Darwin, C. (1872) *The Expression of the Emotions in Man and Animals.* Chicago and London: University of Chicago Press, fifth impression, 1974.

Dunn, J. (1983) 'Sibling relationships in early childhood.' *Child Development 54,* 787–811.

Dunn, J. (1988) 'Annotation: sibling influences on childhood development.' *Journal of Child Psychology and Psychiatry 29,* 2, 119–127.

Dunn, J. and Kendrick, C. (1982) *Siblings: Love, Envy, and Understanding.* London: Grant McIntyre.

Dunn, J. and McGuire, S. (1992) 'Sibling and peer relationships in childhood.' *Journal of Child Psychology and Psychiatry 33,* 1, 67–105.

Ferrari, M. (1984) 'Chronic illness: psychosocial effects on siblings – I. Chronically ill boys.' *Journal of Child Psychology and Psychiatry 25,* 3, 459–476.

Fischer, K.W., Shaver, P.R. and Carnochan, P. (1989) 'A skill approach to emotional development: from basic- to subordinate-category emotions.' In W. Damon (ed) *Child Development Today and Tomorrow.* San Francisco, CA: Jossey-Bass.

Freud, A. (1966) *Normality and Pathology in Childhood: Assessments of Development.* London: Hogarth Press and the Institute of Psycho-Analysis.

Freud, S. (1900) *The Interpretation of Dreams.* Harmondsworth: Penguin, 1976 edition.

Freud, S. (1933) 'Femininity.' In *New Introductory Lectures.* Harmondsworth: Penguin, 1973 edition.

Gesell, A. (1906) 'Jealousy.' *The American Journal of Psychology 17,* 437–496.

Gottlieb, L.N. and Mendelson, M.J. (1990) 'Parental support and firstborn girls' adaptation to the birth of a sibling.' *Journal of Applied Developmental Psychology 11,* 29–48.

Higgins, E.T., Ruble, D.N. and Hartup W.W. (1983) *Social Cognition and Social Development: A Sociocultural Perspective.* Cambridge: Cambridge University Press.

Isaacs, S. (1948) *Children and Parents: Their Problems and Difficulties.* London: Routledge and Kegan Paul, 1968 edition.

Klein, M. (1957) *Envy and Gratitude, and Other Works 1946–1963.* London: Hogarth Press, 1984 impression.

Levy, D.M. (1934) 'Rivalry between children in the same family.' *Child Study 11,* 233–261.

Levy, D.M. (1937) 'Studies in sibling rivalry.' *American Orthopsychiatric Association, Research Monograph, 2.*

McHale, S.M. and Gamble, W.C. (1987) 'Sibling relationships of children with disabled and nondisabled brothers and sisters.' *Developmental Psychology 25,* 3, 421–429.

McKeever, P. (1983) 'Siblings of chronically ill children: a literature review with implications for research and practice.' *American Journal of Orthopsychiatry 53,* 209–218.

Masciuch, S. and Kienapple, K. (1993) 'The emergence of jealousy in children 4 months to 7 years of age.' *Journal of Social and Personal Relationships 10,* 421–435.

Mendelson, M.J. (1990) *Becoming a Brother: A Child Learns About Life, Family, and Self.* Cambridge, Massachusetts and London: MIT Press.

Newman, J. (1994) 'Conflict and friendship in sibling relationships: a review.' *Child Study Journal 24*, 2, 119–154.

Oberndorf, C.P. (1929) 'Psychoanalysis of siblings.' *American Journal of Psychiatry 8*, 1007–20.

Provence, S. and Solnit, A.J. (1983) 'Development-promoting aspects of the sibling experience: vicarious mastery.' *The Psychoanalytic Study of the Child 38*, 337–351.

Robey, K.L., Cohen, B.D. and Epstein, Y.M. (1988) 'The child's response to affection given to someone else: Effects of parental divorce, sex of child, and sibling position.' *Journal of Clinical Child Psychology 17*, 1, 2–7.

Salovey, S.H. and Robey, J. (1984) 'Some antecedents and consequences of social-comparison jealousy.' *Journal of Personality and Social Psychology 47 (4)* 780–792.

Schachter, F.F. and Stone, R.K. (1987) 'Comparing and contrasting siblings: defining the self.' In F.F. Schachter and R.K. Stone (eds) *Practical Concerns About Siblings: Bridging the Research-Practice Gap.* New York and London: The Haworth Press.

Selman, R.L. (1980) *The Growth of Inter-Personal Understanding: Developmental and Clinical Analyses.* New York: Academic Press.

Solnit, A.J. (1983) 'The sibling experience: introduction.' *The Psychoanalytic Study of the Child 38*, 281–284.

Spock, B. (1945) *Baby and Child Care.* 1965 Giant Cardinal edition. New York: Pocket Books.

Stern, D. (1985) *The Interpersonal World of the Infant: A View from Psychoanalysis and Developmental Psychology.* New York: Basic Books.

Stewart, L.H. (1992) *Changemakers: A Jungian Perspective on Sibling Position and Family Atmosphere.* London and New York: Routledge.

Tesser, A. (1980) 'Self-esteem maintenance in family dynamics.' *Journal of Personality and Social Psychology 39*, 77–91.

Vandell, D.L. (1987) 'Baby sister/baby brother: reactions to the birth of a sibling and patterns of early sibling relations.' In F.F. Schachter and R.K. Stone (eds) *Practical Concerns About Siblings: Bridging the Research-Practice Gap.* New York and London: The Haworth Press.

Weisner, T.S. (1982) 'Sibling interdependence and child care-taking: a cross-cultural view.' In M.E. Lamb and B. Sutton-Smith (eds) *Sibling Relationships: Their Nature and Significance Across the Life-Span.* Hillsdale, N.J.: Lawrence Erlbaum Associates.

Winnicott, D.W. (1978) *The Piggle: An Account of the Psycho-Analytical Treatment of a Little Girl.* London: Hogarth Press and the Institute of Psycho-analysis.

# CHAPTER 4

# Troubles of Withdrawal

*Francis Dale*

Children who withdraw – for whatever reasons – from normal social contact pose serious problems for those who are concerned with their welfare whether they be parents, nursery staff, teachers, social workers or medical staff. This is precisely because the symptom itself, withdrawal, makes the task of making contact or communicating with such children – difficult and sometimes impossible.

Frequently, a child shows no interest in other people, rejects all attempts to get close to him/her, and shows no motivation or interest in being helped. To all external appearances, it is other people who have a problem, who are concerned, not the child. As I will attempt to show later, this apparent unconcern on the part of the child is often more perceived than real. It is as if the parents or therapist are required to 'own' the concern for the child and the motivation to do something about it.

In what follows, I will be looking at why children withdraw and the various functions or purposes that it subserves; at the mechanisms or dynamics of withdrawal; and at the impact or effect of withdrawal on both the child and the wider environment. It will also be important to look at different types of withdrawal and how they are influenced by the developmental or maturational stage which the child has attained. Finally, we will look at the different treatment options – based on both a specific and general understanding of the causes of withdrawal in children.

## Why children withdraw

If we exclude children who are withdrawn because of temperamental or constitutional factors, it is probably true to say that the primary aim of withdrawal is avoidance, and further, that avoidance necessarily implies some kind of defence. If we can think of avoidance by withdrawal as a defence, we can then use this knowledge in an investigative way to ask of any particular situation, 'from what threat is the avoidant behaviour protecting the child?'. Once we can formulate a question which relates to a function of withdrawal behaviour, we are in a position to generate hypotheses aimed at seeking its cause(s) and ways of creating the conditions for a successful therapeutic intervention.

### Constitutional/temperamental withdrawal

Some children are described as withdrawn when it would be more accurate to describe them as introverted. The more a society or culture positively values the extraverted, interactive individual, the more likely it is that the introverted child will be seen as 'withdrawn' or 'antisocial'. Sometimes, particularly in large or extended families, the quiet or shy child will be seen as the 'odd one out'. They may themselves feel out of place and socially awkward until they meet someone who understands and respects their need for space and privacy, or become involved in an activity or interest which allows them, and others, to value their more inward-looking natures.

### Reactive withdrawal

This refers to any withdrawal which is in response to an internal or external impingement. An internal impingement could be a physical illness or an emotional or mental preoccupation which re-directs the child's attention or energy inwards and away from the outside. Examples of 'external' impingements might be: hospitalisation, bullying, shock, bereavement, racial discrimination, and varying kinds of physical, sexual, and emotional abuse.

### Psychiatric illness

In childhood, the illnesses which would be most likely to result in the symptom of withdrawal would be: infantile autism, elective mutism, childhood schizophrenia, separation anxiety disorder, eating disorders – especially bulimia and anorexia nervosa – and childhood depression.

### Environmental/socio-cultural withdrawal

Although this heading could be subsumed in the category of reactive withdrawal above, I think it is important enough to merit a heading of its own. For many children, withdrawal is context determined. By this, I am referring to the fact that it is the context in which the child finds him or herself that results in an avoidant behaviour. Hospitalisation has already been mentioned and to this can be added any strange environment that threatens the child's sense of security. Even a previously well adjusted and relatively secure child may show extreme symptoms of withdrawal and depression when faced with the loss of parents and family in an unfamiliar environment (see Wolff 1973).

Withdrawal can also be a reaction to being exposed to a culture that challenges or threatens one's established set of beliefs and attitudes or one's sense of belonging or sense of identity or it can occur in response to racial abuse, religious bigotry or failure to fit in with group norms.

## How children withdraw

The manner in which a child withdraws can be determined by any one of, or a combination of, different factors. The developmental stage the child has reached is one of them.

### Intra-uterine withdrawal

Although the foetus used to be thought of as mindless, insensate and defence-less, empirical data and experimental research has shown this to be untrue. Particularly in the latter stages of pregnancy, the foetus will kick, squirm and turn away from both physical and auditory impingements, avoid bright lights, and try to avoid swallowing a harmless but unpleasant tasting chemical. The foetus has also been shown to be capable of learning a conditioned response to varying kinds of stimuli, the long term effects of which can still be seen in the behaviour of the child after birth. This shows that withdrawal as a means of defending against noxious stimuli, is both present and learned prior to birth.

CLINICAL EXAMPLE (1)

'Alan' was 14 when he was referred to me, along with his parents, to see whether I could help them to understand why he was prone to sudden and frequently violent outbursts of rage and why he had almost totally withdrawn from contact with them apart from eating and sleeping in the family home. Both parents were clearly concerned and at a loss about what they could do to improve the situation. It seemed to me that the intensity and out-of-control nature of Alan's aggressive outbursts was not explicable solely in terms of what was happening in external reality. This suggested that some of his anger, and perhaps the underlying motivation for it, lay elsewhere.

The resolution to the family's dilemma came when I asked the parents when they had first noticed that there was a problem with their son's behaviour. They told me that he had cried non-stop from birth, had wanted to be fed almost continuously, and that he would scream and become intensely distressed if his mother tried to put him down. After nearly two months of this, they were at breaking point and there was the potential for a serious disruption in the relationship between mother and son.

It turned out that when his mother was in the act of delivering him, Alan had been subjected to a life-threatening situation. From it being a normal, problem-free delivery, his mother became distressed, had to be medicated, and was from then on unable to help with the delivery. Alan had to be delivered using forceps. In the process, his head was so distorted that for some days following his birth his parents thought he was brain-damaged.

It is not hard to imagine the impact such a traumatic birth would have had on a newborn baby. From being in a safe, protective environment, where all his primary needs were automatically provided for, Alan would have experienced his birth as a terrifying ordeal – as if he were being dragged out of a safe refuge or sanctuary, attacked, and torn to pieces. It would not be surprising if his parents were not in some way associated with his terrifying ordeal and that at some level he would experience great difficulty in bonding with his mother and being able to relate to her as a loving and protective figure. He might even have felt impelled to protect himself from the mother who had 'attacked' him. One way would have been by withdrawing from her, not trusting her, and in trying to become as self-sufficient and independent as possible given his age and level of maturity. This is in fact exactly what had happened.

When Alan heard this account of his early infantile difficulties and how it could account for the anger he felt towards his parents and his rejection of them, his demeanour immediately changed from a look of intense anger and frustration to one of relief. He at last had an explanation, a way of thinking about and coming to terms with something which, at the time, could not be thought about or resolved.

### The neonate

It should not come as too much of a surprise to learn that we come into the world already primed and equipped to defend ourselves from hostile or unwanted experiences by withdrawal and avoidance. The repertoire may be limited, but it can, nonetheless, be very effective.

In the first weeks, perhaps extending to the first few months, of life, the neonate – being relatively helpless and totally dependent on others for its survival – withdraws mentally and emotionally, using the mechanisms of splitting and projection. Either the unpleasant experience itself or the part of the self which can experience it is split off, disassociated from, or got rid of, and then located somewhere else. If this is not possible then a kind of retreat into the self, into an encapsulated, sealed off inner core, takes place. In this autistic state, the child may appear to be passive, inert, robotic in his movements, unaware of other people, uncommunicative, distant and somehow 'not there'.

The encapsulated autistic state is probably one of the most extreme forms of withdrawal and the most intransigent and resistant to treatment.

### CLINICAL EXAMPLE (2)

John was referred when he was three and a half because of his very demanding, possessive, and controlling behaviour – particularly towards his grandmother. His behaviour was regressive and infantile: he was still in nappies and would not use the toilet; he had screaming tantrums in which he would bite and scratch at his grandmother if she refused him anything; he had no speech, appeared oblivious to verbal instructions, and seemed to live in a world of his own.

He was seen by a child psychotherapist and diagnosed as suffering from autism – a condition in which children withdraw inside themselves, become unreachable, and often exhibit endlessly repetitive, bizarre, and robot-like movements of hands and body.

### THE THERAPY

In the very first session, I had the impression that this child was not 'there' in the room with me. He was present in body but emotionally and mentally he was absent. It soon became clear that, in order to make contact with him, to 'engage' him, I had to change radically the way in which I would normally interrelate with a child in therapy.

Very early on I realised that the only way I could know him and communicate with him was to reach out to him with my attentiveness and to surrender (temporarily) my sense of having a separate identity. At times I had the unnerving experience of losing all sense of bodily awareness apart from my eyes just watching him.

The following extract is from the third session.

John came up to me and put his arms out to me to pick him up. He then put his arms around my neck repeatedly pressing his face and cheeks against mine before lifting his head away to look deeply into my eyes. He began stroking my face with his hands and then put his fingers into his mouth as though he were eating. I commented that he seemed to be wanting to eat me up and have me inside.

Strictly speaking, John was not withdrawn in the sense of being shut inside himself. He was more confused or entangled with people so that, in Frances Tustin's words, 'fragments of the "self" are felt to be dispersed and scattered, so the "self" and "not-self" are inextricably confused' (Tustin 1981).

Therapists working with such children can only really help the child if they understand the child's experience as though it were their own. This is similar to empathy but it is a state which needs to be constantly monitored and the term 'trial identification' (Casement 1985) is perhaps more appropriate. With John, for example, the only way in which I could understand him, was by letting go my sense of separateness and 'letting him in'. It was only later, when I had 'separated myself out' from him that it was possible to think about what had been happening in the session (Dale 1991).

## The young child

Later, however, both physiological and mental maturation allows the young child to develop more sophisticated and complex defences. As the capacity of the ego to mediate between internal demands for immediate satisfaction and the demands of external reality grows, other, less primitive methods of withdrawal become available. As Donald Winnicott – who was that rare animal, a psychoanalyst as well as a paediatrician – found, some children, in response to a failure in infant care, develop what he called a 'false' or compliant self (Winnicott 1976).

Since children who are still totally dependent on their mothers for survival cannot ordinarily choose not to relate to them, they preserve the integrity of what might be called a 'core sense of self' by presenting a compliant self to the world. They react to a – usually – maternal failure to 'recognise', respond to, and to nurture what Winnicott referred to as the 'true-self' of the child, by withdrawing inside. The 'true-self' retreats and becomes encysted or encapsulated and may eventually become out of reach, not only from any meaningful contact with other people – including, and perhaps especially, the parents – but also from the child itself.

CLINICAL EXAMPLE (3)

Patrick entered therapy because his parents found him difficult to cope with. However, apart from complaining of his persistent head banging, they were not able to substantiate this in a convincing way. A careful investigation of their own backgrounds suggested that it was not Patrick's behaviour that caused them difficulty but more what he represented to them internally. Both of them had had very disturbed relations with their parents and both of them had been rejected – the father had been brought up by his grandparents and the mother, while living at home, had been rejected by her father. What they could not tolerate in Patrick was that he somehow reminded them of their own rejection as children. Their response – or defence – was to reject him so that he became the unwanted or objectionable child and not them.

When Patrick first came to see me aged five, he was still living with his parents. Although he was an intelligent and appealing little boy, I was aware that he was holding himself back and only relating to me on the surface. I felt that he only offered people a part of himself and that the core of his personality was shut away somewhere and hidden from view.

Although work was done with Patrick's parents to help them understand why they found him so difficult to tolerate, he was eventually placed with a foster family at their request.

*THE THERAPY*

The main therapeutic work with Patrick has been to provide him with the experience of being in a long-term, consistent and predictable relationship where he can 'be himself' and not have to pretend to be someone or something which he is not. Although it is important to interpret childrens' unconscious fantasies in a manner in which they can understand them, with some children like Patrick the most important element in the therapeutic relationship seems to revolve around your capacity to 'be there for the child'. They do not want you there as a therapist or as an adult but more as a 'real' person who can be there for them, who can think about and experience emotional and mental states which they cannot yet deal with (Dale 1991).

## Withdrawal in the older child

In the older child, the increase in mental and social sophistication allows, in addition to those forms of withdrawal already mentioned, a wider range of options. Perhaps in a similar way to the false-self type of withdrawal where a kind of shell or persona is given the task of relating to the outside while the true self remains hidden away, sometimes it is a part, or a function of the personality like thinking, knowing or feeling that is split off and disassociated from or repressed. If a child is present mentally, then he or she can relate and engage with people in a manner that would be impossible if the feelings appropriate to the thoughts were present. This is similar to what a surgeon needs to do when operating, that is, not to allow emotional responses to interfere with the need to think clearly and objectively. However, in the case of the surgeon, the separation of emotions from thinking is not inappropriate to the situation and neither is it pathological – it is ego syntonic. That is, it is a proper use of ego functioning in relation to the demands of external reality, and not using the ego to avoid or withdraw from reality.

There are other kinds of partial withdrawal: for example, having minimal contact with parents or teachers whilst spending every available minute with one's friends; or channelling all of one's energy into a specialised interest or pursuit like stamp collecting, bird watching, fishing, chess, music, reading and so on.[1] More worrying forms of withdrawal are when a child retreats into a private fantasy world which is not shared by anyone else, or takes drugs.

---

1    I am not suggesting that everyone who engages in these pursuits is doing so in order to withdraw from social contact.

A healthier form of withdrawal relates to any activity or interest where the withdrawal is not away from contact with others, so much as a re-direction of libido – mental energy – into a subjective, intense preoccupation with one's inner world. One finds this kind of withdrawal or sublimation predominantly in artistic people: painters, writers, musicians and poets. Children who would fall into this category would be those who are highly intelligent or gifted in some way. 'Linda', an elective mute girl whom I will be talking about later, falls into this latter category although there were other factors that combined to make her withdrawal a pathological one.

## Consequences of withdrawal

One of the main problems of withdrawal is that, while it may protect the child, at the same time it isolates and distances him from being able to communicate about his predicament or to respond easily to help that is available. In other words, the symptom itself continues and augments a dysfunctional response to others. This varies of course depending on the level of pathology involved in the withdrawal. However, if we take an extreme case of withdrawal, the autistic child – such as 'John' – it becomes clear that protection or defence of the self results in having no self, of being isolated, encapsulated in inner space and unable or unwilling to make contact with others.

Another consequence of withdrawal is the sense of helpless frustration and impotence that is evoked in those who are involved in any way with the child. For parents, it can result in an overwhelming sense of despair and guilt. They feel at fault, responsible in some way but without knowing why or what can be done to remedy the situation. In some situations, the child has withdrawn in order to punish the parent(s). This can result in the parents feeling full of rage and frustrated impotence, leading them to to retaliate and reject the child in turn. It can also draw out sadistic responses in the parents who experience the child's withdrawal as a personal attack. In this circumstance, the parents feel punished and humiliated by their child's lack of responsiveness. They may eventually react to the child's continual rejection of their love and care by turning against him or her in an aggressive, even taunting way. They seek not only to return the rejection they experience by rejecting the child but also to return the 'attack' that they feel the withdrawal to be.

In the school situation, teaching staff may either not notice the child because he or she poses no overtly difficult or stressful behaviour patterns, or feel like the parents, frustrated, impotent and useless. In either case, the education of the child may suffer – either in a purely educational sense, or socially by severely restricting his interaction with his peers.

CLINICAL EXAMPLE (4)

'Michael' was born with an allergy to his mother's milk. He became severely malnourished and was admitted to hospital at six weeks of age and fed on a drip for two weeks. Following this, he had to be fed on a special milk diet but was clearly very disturbed, being impossible to comfort and crying almost continuously for the first six months of life.

He was referred to a Child Guidance clinic when he was eight because he seemed to be unhappy and isolated, and because of his outbursts of temper which were mainly directed at his brother who was only ten and a half months younger than him. There are several obvious similarities between Michael's neonatal trauma and that of Alan's. Both responded in similar ways: inconsolable crying and distress and violent episodes of rage.

*THE THERAPY*

Michael presented as a very stiff, even rigid boy, with a serious expression and a peculiarly empty, almost 'shell-like' quality to him. He was restless, had poor concentration, few friends and seemed to live in a world of his own. In exploring his early history it became apparent that the relationship between Michael and his mother had never really recovered from the traumatic separation which took place when he had to go into hospital. His mother felt that she had never been able to get as close to him as she had to his brother.

As with other cases of early infantile trauma, the damage had occurred at a time in Michael's development before he had developed a capacity to think or to process what had happened to him. His mother's absence during those two weeks meant that she was not available to take on board and manage his anxiety for him. Two weeks in a baby's life is probably an eternity. By the time he returned home, his sense of trust in his mother's capacity to protect and care for him must have been severely damaged. The birth of his brother so soon afterwards, and the experience of seeing his brother feed successfully at his mother's breast, must have been the final blow to any attempts he may have made at rebuilding the broken relationship between himself and his mother.

An early focus in therapy, therefore, was to try to heal the rift between mother and child by encouraging her to explain to Michael as an eight year old what had happened and why when he was a baby. The aim of this was to create a 'benign split'[2] in Michael between the baby part of him which

---

2  A 'benign split' refers to a process whereby the therapist or patient is able to differentiate an observing part of the personality which is then capable of thinking without being taken over by unconscious processes.

had not been able to understand or cope with what had happened to him and the more grown up part which now could (Dale 1991).

## Communicating with the withdrawn child

If I can use a metaphor to illustrate the wrong kind of approach to establishing rapport or trust with the withdrawn child, it would be to picture a hermit crab that has retreated into its shell being encouraged out by someone poking and prodding at it with a stick. Adopting a direct – and particularly, a confrontational attitude – with a withdrawn child is likely to make matters worse rather than better. An indirect approach, and one which, furthermore, respects the need of the child both to remain in control and maintain his or her personal boundaries, is much more likely to succeed in drawing the child out and establishing a basis for a trusting relationship.

I think there is a tendency amongst some professionals whose primary training and expertise is not geared to one-to-one work with children to assume that the child's agenda will be the same as their own and that children are 'little adults' who basically feel and think about the world in the same way that they do. I think these are dangerous and incorrect assumptions to hold about children – particularly those whose experience has taught them to be wary of adults.

In my experience, the most effective way to make contact with a withdrawn child is to try to identify empathically with him, to try and understand, from the child's perspective, how he feels about coming to see you and what anxieties, wishes, or fantasies he has. In the beginning, it is far better spending time getting to know the child and making a connection with him, than in asking lots of questions. If you establish a relationship with the child and take an interest in him, the questions – and the answers to them – will emerge naturally and usually spontaneously out of the interaction between yourself and the child.

There are several factors which can have a positive or negative influence on our ability to enter into a therapeutic relationship with the child, but the most important of these is our ability to respect the personal boundaries of the child. For example, if we are a familiar and trusted figure, or someone whose role makes us safe (close relative, teacher, health visitor, nurse or doctor), then the child will feel less threatened or intimidated than if we are a relatively unknown figure (although even doctors and nurses can be frightening figures as we shall see later).

In the latter case, we may need to be more circumspect in approaching the child in order to give him or her sufficient time to 'get the feel of us' and to weigh up whether we are a safe or a threatening figure.

The younger the child, the more dependent they are on their carers, the less secure in their basic relationships, the more unfamiliar the environment (for example, a child will feel less anxious if confronted by a stranger when on his or her own territory), the more anxious they will be in an unfamiliar situation and the more in need of reassurance (Dale 1991).

Perhaps the most important factor in communicating with the withdrawn child is our capacity to observe and make use of non-verbal forms of communication. We can see how important this is for without it mothers would have no means of making sense of, and hence being able to respond to, their babies' primitive attempts to communicate.

Anyone who has watched a mother interacting with her baby will know that the communication between the mother and child is mainly taking place at a non-verbal level. While the *content* of what the mother is saying may be meaningless from a rational point of view one can see that the baby is being effectively communicated to and that he does feel understood.

Many mothers will tell you – although they may not be able to rationalise it – that they know what their baby is feeling: whether he is sad, angry, puzzled, frightened, confused, hungry, uncomfortable, in pain, falling apart, contented, ecstatic or blissful. They probably cannot explain how they know because this kind of 'knowing' is not a cognitive process. It is an understanding which is conveyed by way of impact, by the emotional resonance that someone we are relating to has on us. While this is an unconscious process, there are ways in which we can learn to recognise when this is happening.

The first thing to understand is that in all relationships, whether we are aware of it or not, we are continually being affected by, and responding to, the emotional and mental states of the people we are relating to. The mother knows what the baby is feeling because she experiences the emotional state of the baby as though it were her own.

Thus, if her baby panics or experiences intense anxiety, she experiences – if only for a moment – the same emotion (she will become overwhelmed by panic, or filled with anxiety). On the other hand, if the baby is blissfully contented, she shares in that state too. What this shows us is that there is a form of communication or interaction between individuals which exists alongside, and which is independent of, verbal communication.

This clearly has important implications in our therapeutic work with withdrawn children, many of whom we can only understand by becoming conscious of the emotional impact they have on us (Dale 1991).

## Treating the withdrawn child

In the clinical examples above, I have given some examples of different ways of thinking about and treating the withdrawn child and his family. John, the autistic boy, had probably become withdrawn due to his mother's abandonment of him at an early age; Alan and Michael both reacted in the same way to early birth/postnatal trauma by distancing themselves from their parents; and Patrick hid away from any meaningful contact with people behind a 'false-self' personality structure.

I would now like to give some other examples of therapy with children who, for a variety of reasons, have become withdrawn.[3]

## Psychotic withdrawal

Some forms of withdrawal in children are based on either the terror of complete annihilation or disintegration, or on the fear of persecutory attacks from malevolent forces. Frequently, there is little or no 'healthy' or integrated part of the child's personality which one can relate to. In the presence of such children, one can often feel that they are 'not there', that there is 'nobody at home'. Alternatively, people who come into contact with such children may feel that they are not there for the child.

Although therapy with such severely damaged children can be exceedingly difficult and drawn out, they can sometimes be rescued if one can persevere and tolerate the long periods when no apparent progress is being made (Dale 1991).

### CLINICAL EXAMPLE (5)

Sundip was referred because his teachers were becoming concerned at his increasingly bizarre behaviour and social isolation. Due to his hysterical reactions when anyone made an approach to him, he was mercilessly bullied and teased at school. He wrote the following comments in an exam:

> God needed a prison, so he created the Earth ... Thunder is when God is angry with the whole of a small area and stamps his feet, rain and snow are when he is furious with a very large area... After such a punishment as the Earth nobody commits any more sins in Heaven ... Life is a sentence, so I hope I die soon. (Dale 1984)

From the very first meeting, Sundip regarded me with undisguised suspicion and hostility. Whenever I tried to engage him with an interpretation he would become quite paranoid and shout and talk in a very penetrating high-pitched voice, jumping up and down and waving his arms and threatening to tell his mother all about me and my lies...this sort of omnipotent and

---

3    The following clinical examples also appear in my chapter in *Truants From Life* published by David Fulton, 1991.

controlling behaviour left me feeling as if I were constantly on a knife edge with him and that the success or failure of therapy hung literally by a thread. However, in spite of living with the constant fear that either therapy or Sundip would break down…some cracks in his very brittle defences began to appear. This started with Sundip repeatedly asking me what 'therapy' was and 'how it worked' and wanting to know what the perentage of successes to failures was… I gradually began to realise that despite his dread of me and what I might do to him, nothing could be worse than being where he was already. As therapy opened up the floodgates of what seemed to be a boundless reservoir of misery, I began at last to feel a faint ray of hope (Dale 1984).

Both Sundip and John – the autistic boy already referred to – needed to be seen in more intensive therapy in order to contain the anxiety that coming out of their isolation caused them. In both cases, their defence was 'not to know', to split off or deny any awareness that would reveal what it was that they could not confront *inside themselves*. What differentiated them from the other children we have previously discussed was the intensity of the affect they generated in their therapist, their failure to adapt to the demands of external reality, and their inability to maintain and defend an *integrated* personality structure from being overwhelmed and fragmented by pathological processes.

## Elective mutism

CLINICAL EXAMPLE (6)

'Linda' was ten when she was referred to me because, apart from her mother, and to a lesser extent her father, she was almost totally mute. If she spoke at all, it was either through her mother – in which case she would furtively whisper into her ear – or by way of written messages. She never looked at anyone and avoided any eye contact.

In school, she was totally silent and would only communicate to the teachers through one or two of the other girls in the class who would speak for her. She was, however, very artistic and probably gifted. She had written a poem of such quality and maturity that both teachers and fellow pupils were amazed and she had also produced artwork and drawings of a very high standard.

In the whole of the eighteen months that I saw Linda on a once-weekly basis, she only spoke to me once and that was to ask me what my birth date was. She would come into the room where I saw her, sit down with her head bowed and hair hanging down so that her face was hidden from view and immediately begin to draw. At the end of the session, she would put her things away and get up and leave without once having looked at me.

Her drawings were remarkable – both for the speed with which she executed them, and for the artistic talent she displayed. Whilst she may have been withdrawn on the outside, on the 'inside', she revealed a liveliness, versatility, curiosity and fine intelligence which were ordinarily completely hidden from view. She also displayed a very contemptuous and denigrating attitude towards me which only changed when I was able to interpret her wish to know my birth sign as a means of getting to know about me without having to reveal anything of herself.

Although Linda refused to talk to people, she did want to relate to them – but on her terms. She had an extraordinary knowledge of astrology, knowing by heart all of the astrological signs, their dates, symbolic representations, their compatibility with each other, the characteristics of personality associated with each sign and much else besides.

By knowing my birth sign she could almost 'do away with me' because she could metaphorically 'get inside me' without having to relate to me at all 'on the outside'. The sense of omniscience and power which this gave her was used in a very destructive way to devalue what other people had to offer. If she could get inside them and know all about them – even things they did not know about themselves – then she did not need them, could do without them and, as it were, feed off her own internal resources.

Over a period of months it was possible to build up a picture of her internal world based almost entirely on the drawings which she produced in our sessions together. These revealed the existence of an inner life which was in total contrast to the extremely shy, withdrawn and rather insipid child that she presented to the world.

Her drawings were colourful and vibrant, and full of powerful and evocative imagery mainly drawn from her extensive knowledge of fairy stories and folk tales. These were full of allusions to the themes of sexuality, romance and jealousy and revealed how preoccupied she was by her developing sexuality and the problem of giving expression to it safely.

When Linda made the transition to secondary school, although still not talking to me, she was relating to me much more openly through the medium of her drawings which had in any case become her way of talking to me. In her new school she was able to come out of herself more, establish a close circle of friends and seemed happy and well integrated.

## Traumatic separation
CLINICAL EXAMPLE (7)

Steven was eighteen months old when he was rushed to hospital after he tripped and crashed through a glass coffee-table. He sustained the most horrific injuries to his upper palate and lip and had nearly bled to death. He could still remember the accident and his terror when he had to be held down while the surgeon stitched up the gaping wound to his face... When he was seventeen, he became completely obsessed with the thought that he was going to die and had panic attacks in which he would feel as if he were suffocating.

He presented as a very intense, serious and agitated young man whose body was so full of nervous energy that he could not keep still for more than a few minutes at a time. In addition to his fear of dying, he complained about feeling 'out of place' and not being understood or accepted by fellow students at the college where he was studying.

Steven's defence against being overwhelmed by anxiety was to deny the significance of anything which could not be explained on a purely rational basis. While this protected him from the irrational and unconscious aspects of his mental life, it also left him feeling empty and impoverished.

Trying to help Steven get in touch with his feelings and unconscious anxieties was made all the more difficult not only because of his need to over-intellectualise everything but also because, his feeling life having been denied for so long, he experienced any contact with his emotions as dangerous and persecuting. If I made any interpretations which threatened to reveal something about himself which he did not know of, he would become extremely agitated and defensive, and dismissive, even contemptuous, of me.

What I learned of Steven's family life further reinforced the view that being in touch with one's feelings was dangerous. For some reason, Steven's mother had never successfully bonded with him as a baby. However, she was able to form a close emotional bond with his sister who had been born just before his accident. He was closer to his father but there were tensions between his parents which had resulted in a split between mother and daughter on one side and father and son on the other. Steven described his mother as distant, cold and unemotional and remarked that his father had had a breakdown at the same age he was now, and that as a young man *he also* had had fears of dying.

However, in spite of Steven's ambivalence regarding therapy – seeing it as much as a threat as a help – his capacity to make links between what had happened to him in hospital, his current fear of dying, and the way his family denied emotions, made it possible for him to be able to understand his anxieties both as an expression of unresolved terrors from his early childhood and pathological patterns of relating in the family.

CLINICAL EXAMPLE (8)

Malcolm suffered from a rare congenital deformity in which one half of his body, including the bones in his head, had developed assymetrically. By the age of seven, he was having to wear a built-up shoe and the bones of one whole side of his body were noticeably smaller than those of the other side. He was admitted to hospital where the long bone in his thigh was cut in half and gradually pulled apart over a period of months in order to encourage extra bone growth. He spent the best part of a year in hospital and although his parents visited him regularly, he felt abandoned by them and would go into blind panics and tantrums when they attempted to leave after visits.

After leaving hospital he had to wear a plaster cast which came up to his waist, could not go to the toilet unaided and had to be pushed around the playground and to and from the school in a pram.

Malcolm was referred for therapy at the age of fifteen because of 'difficulties in coping with life'. However, he was completely unable to explain the nature of these problems to his doctor except to say that for the past two years he had been 'preoccupied with thoughts of life and the workings of the mind' and was unable to distinguish at times between reality and fantasy. He was very conscious that his body was different from other peoples' and avoided situations where this might be noticed. This meant that he never joined in with his peers in gymnastics, games or any competitive sports.

As with Steven, it proved very difficult to make contact with him at anything other than an intellectual level. The following extract from an early session is fairly typical of the confused and convoluted way his 'thinking' blocked any attempts at understanding.

Malcolm began by saying that he had these troubles.

I wondered if he could tell me about them.

He replied that he just couldn't stop thinking about world problems.

Were there any problems in particular that bothered him? No. He just felt that he had 'this problem' which he had always to think about and that thinking about it stopped him from concentrating.

I again wondered if he could try and tell me a little more about this problem which he had to keep thinking about.

He responded by saying that there were times when he could be distracted by something which interested him but then he would realise that he had not been thinking about 'his problem' and would not be able to remember anything and his mind would go blank and he would panic. (Dale 1983)

After several sessions like this one my mind was becoming blank. I was confused, could not think clearly, was losing track of what was going on in the session and becoming increasingly frustrated. What I failed to realise at the time was how much I may have been experiencing in the countertransference Malcolm's own confused state of mind. It was also a very powerful attack on my thinking. When I was able to point out to him how his thinking capacity was being used in a very destructive way in order to prevent understanding and not to promote it, the underlying cause of his present difficulties – his catastrophic experience in hospital as a child – began to emerge. Little by little we were able to build up a picture of what it had been like for Malcolm to be taken away from family, friends, school – a familiar environment – and to be subjected to various traumatic surgical procedures, to have to lie on his back in traction for nearly a year. It became very clear in therapy that he had experienced the ministrations of the doctors and nurses not as helpful but as an assault or invasion on his person in which he was a passive and defenceless victim at the mercy of cruel and sadistic persecutors.

As therapy progressed, Malcolm began to get in touch – on a more conscious level – with the damaged child he was still carrying inside, so that he became increasingly able to relate to people and situations in the here and now and less in terms of his earlier experiences. (Dale 1983)

Finally, I would like to share another case, like Patrick's above, where the withdrawn behaviour seemed to be specifically connected to a lack of attachment or a failure of the mother to bond with the child in infancy.

## Withdrawal and lack of attachment

CLINICAL EXAMPLE (9)

I began seeing Peter when he was seven years old. As a baby, he had been virtually abandoned by his natural mother who used to leave him in his pram to scream and cry for hours on end. He was eventually taken into care at six months of age and was adopted when he was 18 months old.

When I first saw Peter he was a very silent, withdrawn and angry child. As with Linda, he communicated almost entirely through his drawings.

He rarely if ever spoke to me, and when he did it was usually to denigrate or mock something which I had just interpreted to him. He did, however, always listen very carefully to the comments I made about his drawings and these became, from the very first session, his preferred way of having a dialogue with me.

Peter's contempt for me was really an expression of the hatred and anger which he felt over his abandonment by his parents, projected onto me. It was also I think, a very primitive way of getting rid of his own sense of not being wanted, of being rubbished and deeply wounded.

Peter needed me to know what it must have been like to be rubbished and rejected in this way – in the way in which he must have felt rubbished as a child. He needed more than this of course; he also needed to know that

I was *prepared to hold onto these feelings and dangerous thoughts for him*, and not only to survive them, but also understand and make sense of them.

Peter never openly acknowledged that he got anything out of coming to see me. But he never missed a session – and in his drawings, he showed that he was influenced by my understanding of what was happening inside of him and between us.

Most of the withdrawn children I have seen over the years have been very adept at getting other people to experience the frustration and rejection which they found it so difficult to accept themselves. Many of them have long ago given up trying to relate to other people, and in their frustration and hurt have responded to attempts to get through to them by behaving in a hostile, rejecting and punishing way that leaves parents, teachers, friends and therapists feeling bruised, baffled, useless and angry.

Such rejection is based on sadism but a sadism not only directed against the therapist but also unconsciously against the vulnerable and dependent part of the child which the therapist is seen as representing.

It is precisely because these children can make people feel so useless and devalued that one has to resist retaliating by rejecting them in return. I often felt like giving up on Peter but I knew that if I did it would be 'acting out' on my part and not based on therapeutic considerations. The ability of the therapist to be able to bear and 'contain' (both emotionally and cognitively) such difficult emotions gradually helps the child to be able to do this for himself.

An important factor which one needs to take into account when working with disturbed children, and one which frequently is not given enough attention, is the impact that working with such children can have on the therapist, teacher or health professional. It is easier to notice this with children who are overtly angry or distressed but much more difficult when the child is withdrawn and does not 'act out' in such an obvious manner.

However, as the following quotes demonstrate, the demands on the therapist's capacity to manage – even to survive – 'difficult to bear states' is central to the successful outcome of therapeutic work with such children:

> She made me know *in myself* [my italics] what it was like to be excluded, discarded and shut out. Suddenly I would find myself experiencing extraordinary anger which I felt to be, in part at least, a projection of her own feelings... I was to be rendered useless by her attacks on my capacity to think about and understand her pain.

> He had a numb, unreachable quality which the therapist found very hard to get through... This brick-wall quality was very hard to penetrate and, although expressed differently, had a quality of forceful projection of

unpleasant and painful feelings into the therapist. (Boston and Szur 1983)

It seems then that these children are so difficult to approach, not just because they have withdrawn themselves from normal contact, but because the contact they need to make with us can only be experienced through what they make us feel.

They need us to have their painful feelings, their emptiness and despair, to be able to tolerate and think about and contain these states for them until they feel safe enough to be able to do this for themselves (Dale 1991).

## References

Boston, M. and Szur, R. (1983) (eds) *Psychotherapy with Severely Deprived Children*. London: Routledge and Kegan Paul.

Casement, P. (1985) *On Learning From the Patient*. London: Tavistock.

Dale, F. (1983) 'The body as bondage: work with two children with physical handicap.' *Journal of Child Psychotherapy 9*, 1.

Dale, F. (1984) 'The re-unification of Sundip: the bringing together of split-off parts of the personality in a boy with psychotic features.' *Journal of Child Psychotherapy 10*, 2.

Dale, F. (1991) 'The art of communicating with vulnerable children.' In V. Varma (ed) *The Secret Life of Vulnerable Children*. London: Routledge.

Dale, F. (1991) 'The psychotherapeutic treatment of withdrawn children.' In V. Varma (ed) *Truants From Life*. London: David Fulton Publishers.

Tustin, F. (1981) *Autistic States in Children*. London: Routledge and Kegan Paul.

Winnicott, D. (1976) *The Maturational Processes and the Facilitating Environment*. London: The Hogarth Press and the Institute of Psycho-Analysis.

Wolff, S. (1973) *Children Under Stress*. Harmondsworth: Penguin.

CHAPTER 5

# Troubles of Aggressiveness

*Francis Dale*

There probably has never been – nor ever will be – a society or culture in which aggressiveness does not exist in some form or other. While it may be debatable whether we have a specific instinct for aggression, without it the human race would not survive. In modern day society, we succeed or fail by way of competitiveness, self-interest, whether personal, familial or national, as well as through the aggressive assertion of our rights, just as in the past we succeeded by wielding the axe, the spear and the sword. Even if we as individuals are not physically aggressive, other people take on that role on our behalf. If someone threatens us, we call the police; if another power tries to dominate or coerce, we call in the troops. It is not aggression itself that is the problem but rather, how it is employed, for what purpose, and whether it is an appropriate response to the situation in which it is used as the primary means of resolving an issue. In what follows, we will be looking at why children and adolescents turn to aggression to resolve issues, the circumstances in which aggression is likely to be elicited, the ways in which it is manifested and communicated, and, finally, how it can be handled and understood.

## Why children turn to aggression

### Frustration

Frustration is perhaps the most frequent cause of aggression in babies and young children. Whenever a primary or instinctual need is withheld for longer than the baby or small child can tolerate, at some point an aggressive reaction is an almost inevitable outcome. There are several reasons for this but they all revolve around the relative developmental immaturity of the small child. The primary cause of frustration in babies is loss of contact with the breast. Early on, this is not experienced by the baby as merely 'loss of the breast', but more as the psychic equivalent to the loss of the mother–baby unit, or the state of being in an *undifferentiated at-oneness* with the mother (Mahler, Pine and Bergman 1987).

For the first few months of life, the mother – or more accurately the mother as breast – is not clearly differentiated from the self. All good experiences derive from an ongoing identification with the self as breast. Any premature disruption of this identity, or union with the 'breast as self', can lead to the baby experiencing the breast which is at this stage emotionally and psychically equivalent to the mother as a whole person, as 'not self' (Tustin 1981).

In order to begin the long process of individuation, which involves an increasing capacity to deal with external reality or 'not self' experiences, at some stage the baby needs to be able to differentiate between the illusion of the breast and self as one, and the self as being in relationship with the mother or breast as a *separate* and *autonomous person*. However, if this happens too early – before the baby's ego can cope with the knowledge of the mother's separateness – then the baby will feel overwhelmed by catastrophic, disintegrative states which cannot be thought about, processed or experienced. In this situation, the 'absent' breast is experienced as a *persecuting presence* as well as 'not self'. Subjectively, this is experienced as an aggressive and destructive attack on the self and has to be defended against. The baby's aggression will be mobilised and expressed in a variety of ways: screaming, fretting, extreme restlessness and agitated movements, biting the nipple and the violent expulsion of bodily products such as faeces, urine and food. (In the first few months of life the self is experienced in a somato-sensory way in which bodily products are concretely equated with mental or emotional states. Thus, defecation can be the bodily equivalent to getting rid of bad parts of the self.)

As the self and 'object' (i.e. breast or mother) become more clearly differentiated from each other, the baby can tolerate 'not self' experiences for longer periods and with less catastrophic results. The young child can use its own body auto-erotically to lessen the damaging effects of 'not self' experiences and, in fantasy, by resorting to hallucinatory gratification where the child uses 'magical thinking' to create or mould its experience into the shape it requires. When the child sucks his thumb, he is, in a very concrete way, creating a somato-sensory experience which, in fantasy, can replace the breast. He is now not so absolutely dependent on the mother to provide for all of his needs. He can, both in reality and in fantasy, meet some of his needs himself.

However, this awareness that he can meet some of his needs himself can in turn lead to a different form of frustration. The very awareness that allows him to see his mother as separate also reveals to him, in a way that was not possible before, the true extent of his dependency. While there are some things he can do for himself, he becomes increasingly aware of just how much he cannot do. Throughout childhood, stages are reached which provide satisfaction and competence at one level whilst simultaneously confronting the child with the realisation of how much he cannot do and the true extent of his dependence on his parents. The anger which the child may express in the forms of temper tantrums, obstinacy and disobedience, results from the tension between the realisation of its dependency on its parents, and the omnipotent wish to be in control, to be self sufficient and autonomous.

### Fear

After frustration, fear is a common cause of aggression. The 'fight or flight' response is an instinctual reaction to situations where there is perceived to be an immediate threat to the organism. If flight or escape is not possible, animals will often react with extremely hostile and aggressive behaviour (Lorenz 1970). Children – and babies even more so – are not usually in a position to defend themselves realistically against threats to their emotional, mental or physical well-being. In normal circumstances, they rely on their parents to do this for them. Problems arise when for whatever reason the protective function of the parents fails. If the protective shield placed around the child by the parents fails from time to time, then, depending on the degree of threat involved and the ego strength of the child, the hostile feelings evoked by the threat will not be experienced as too dangerous or destructive. Frequently, however – as already pointed out above – the source of threat is perceived as coming from the parents themselves. When this is the case, it is frequently difficult – if not impossible – to express openly the hostile impulses engendered towards one's parent(s).

The hostile impulses can be dealt with in a variety of ways. In the very young child, before a functioning ego as such has developed, repressing aggressive or hostile impulses is not possible. There has to be some differentiation between psychic structures – between a conscious ego-self and an unconscious – before repression can occur. They can, however, be 'split' or fragmented. Hostile impulses, and the part of the self which can experience them, can be got rid of, displaced, and projected elsewhere. If these aggressive impulses can be projected into an object or person (usually the parent) who can contain, detoxify, and manage them, then the fear of the damage done to the object – the breast, mother, father etc. – is not experienced as overwhelming or as evoking retaliation from whoever the hostile impulses has projected into. If the child's aggressive impulses can be contained, thought about and detoxified in this way over time, then gradually he or she becomes identified with, or internalises, a 'parental model' for dealing with aggression effectively and safely.

If, however, the child does not meet a good enough container for its hostile impulses, the splitting does not become modified and over time replaced by more effective, mature and reality-based solutions and a pathological response to aggression sets in. In this case, aggression may be dealt with either by turning it in on the self, or projecting it outwards.

## Aggression turned inwards

Aggressive impulses are turned in on the self when it is felt to be too dangerous – either to oneself or to others we care about – to express them openly. Frequently, the child's aggressive impulses cannot be tolerated by the child, either because those parental figures upon whom it is totally dependent for survival would feel too threatened by them, or because of the fear of punishment and retaliation. For some children, their experience of their parents as containers is similar to being totally dependent on a lifebelt which barely keeps your head out of the water. If even the smallest wave threatens to push you under, you cannot risk doing anything which threatens the precarious stability of your lifebelt. When a parent or carer is experienced as the equivalent of a 'leaky' lifebelt, the child may have no option but to protect him or her from his aggression or hostility. The parent is not 'buoyant' enough to contain the child's aggression (or any difficult-to-bear emotion) in a safe enough way. In the above situation, it is both easier and safer to punish the self. An 'attack' on the self is survivable, an attack on a leaky lifebelt is not.

Aggression which is turned in on the self is frequently rationalised in terms of an unconscious sense of guilt. The child believes he must be bad because his parents do not love him, treat him badly, punish or ignore him. Therefore he *deserves* to be punished. This then provides the rationale for the child to take control of the punishment. He does this because he has no option and because it fits in with his belief system. The most primitive form of self-punishment is expressed through the body by way of somatisation or self-harm. Headaches or migraine, stomach upsets, back pain, asthma, eczema and boils can all be physiological responses to anger which cannot be thought about.


## Displaced or projected aggression

There are basically two ways in which hostile impulses can be got rid of through projection. The most common – and in terms of pathology, the most 'healthy' – is by *scapegoating*. In scapegoating, someone, or some*thing*, is chosen as a receptacle or focus for receiving aggressive impulses. Anyone who has been so unwise as to interfere in a family or marital dispute will be familiar with the experience of finding that the person(s) on whose behalf you intervened can suddenly turn on you as though you were the common enemy. What has happened is that *you* have become the scapegoat and become a focus for the aggression which was formerly directed elsewhere.

Aggression which is displaced in this way is always a sign of a failure in the capacity to 'contain', to process or think about it in a more ego syntonic way. This is why, in general, children choose to displace or project their hostile impulses more than adults. Their egos have not yet learned how to deal with aggression effectively. They learn how to do this by modelling or identifying with their parental models. If they have poor parental models, then they will not be able to internalise, or identity with, an effective model for dealing with aggression.

Another, more pathological way of dealing with aggression, is through *identification with the aggressor*. In his moving and disturbing book about concentration camps, *Man's Search for Meaning* (1969), Viktor Frankl talks about the various strategies that his fellow inmates adopted in order to increase their chances of survival – not just physically but also mentally, emotionally and spiritually. Certain individuals became 'Capos'. These were ordinary inmates who *chose* to become camp guards – responsible for work details, distribution of food, organising the daily routine and also for the awarding of special favours or considerations and the meting out of punishments. Some of them would even attempt to wear military style uniforms and ape the arrogance and brutishness of the S.S. guards. In identifying with the aggressor, they become like him, they adopted his attitudes, his belief systems, certain ruthless traits of personality and, most importantly, they became powerful, strong and in control. *They* were now the aggressors and other people the weak, powerless, impotent and terrified victims. Psychologically, they had reversed their situation. However, at another level, they were also attacking the helpless, vulnerable part of themselves, now *projected into someone else*. This is a very destructive cycle for a child (or adult) to get into. They are not only using someone else as a dustbin into whom they can dump unwanted parts of themselves which can then be disparaged or attacked, but they risk losing touch with a part or aspect of themselves which needs their help and understanding.

### Loss of love

Studies of attachment in the human infant have provided very strong evidence for the crucial importance of bonding on the infant's well-being (Bowlby 1972). Any disruption or premature disturbance to the bond between the mother and child is experienced as a threat to its very existence. As pointed out above, the early relationship between mother and infant is one where there is very little awareness of separation. Being loved and being at one with the mother are probably psychically equivalent states of being. Any loss of, or threat to, the state of undifferentiated at-oneness with the mother will, therefore, be resisted with all the resources at the infant's disposal. One of these is aggression. The baby is limited in the ways in which it can express aggression: it can scream, explosively evacuate its bowels, vomit, bite, or violently throw itself about. Much of its aggression – and distress – is somatised. That is, it is expressed not symbolically through words, but concretely through its body language. Perhaps all aggression in babies is ultimately connected to the loss of the loved object

– initially the breast (part object), then the mother (whole object), and later the father.

Because the baby cannot survive without its primary attachment figure, the hostility which it feels towards it when there is a threat to its attachment to it, has to be disguised or denied in some way. 'Splitting' the object so that the 'bad' part is kept separate from the 'good' part is one option. This type of defence allows hostile impulses to be expressed without the baby being overwhelmed with anxiety at having destroyed the good and loving relationship in the process. However, if this splitting becomes habitual, hateful impulses cannot become modified by loving impulses, and the relationship to the 'good' object becomes false (Winnicott 1976). It becomes false because it is dominated by the need to keep aggressive impulses – and the part of the self which experiences them – hidden. This also results in an impoverishment of the self and a shallowness of affect. Frequently, you will hear parents of children who have developed problems in later life saying '…but he/she was such a *good* baby'. These children never cause any problems because they have learned to hide or deny them. The parents' love was not felt to be strong enough to survive the anger at unmet needs and loss of love.

Older children, who are both more solidly attached to their parental figures, and more separate and individuated, can own their anger and hostility more openly. When there is a withdrawal of love, they can more readily react with anger because they know from experience that the love they have for their parents – and vice versa – will survive. They also have another mechanism for dealing with loss and anger that was absent before – language. The mother or father can now provide the child with explanations which help the child deal with frustration, uncertainty and anxiety. Thinking, which is impossible without language, provides the child with a means for resolving, curtailing, attenuating, rationalising or denying anger, other than just acting it out. It stands to reason, therefore, that children who have been brought up in families where anger is rarely resolved through debate or understanding do not internalise a model where anger can be modified through thought. It has to be got rid of, expelled, pushed into someone else.

## When children turn to aggression

Having looked at the 'why' of aggression, it is now time to look at the 'when' of aggression. Aggression is never arbitrary. It has a cause, an aim or function, a focus and a particular mode of expression. Because aggression is sometimes displaced or denied it is not always easy to ascertain either the cause or the focus. By asking the question, 'Why now?' one can begin to look for correlations between the anger and the context in which it manifests itself. Although the context may be in the present, its roots may derive from much earlier events.

In other words, anger in the here and now, and the context in which it appears, allow us to make deductions concerning its genetic roots. Let me give you an example.

A family decided to have a treat and go out for a meal. The father became aware almost as soon as he sat down in the restaurant that he was feeling anxious. His children – who were normally very well behaved – began to bicker (he realised later that they had probably been affected by his inner tension). His daughter was then brought a drink by a waitress which was so full that it was almost brimming over the edge of the glass. Although it was almost inevitable that the drink would be spilled, when it was, the father felt embarrassed, tense and angry. He knew with his head, that it was an 'accident waiting to happen' but his mood became worse and he left the restaurant before the meal was finished. Once he had left the restaurant, his irritability and moodiness left him. However, later that same day, he realised that he was depressed and tried to make sense of it. He felt that it was connected in some way with the incident earlier in the day when his daughter had spilled the drink. Then it came to him.

When he was one and a half years old, his mother had to go into hospital and he was placed in an orphanage run by nuns. His father had died fairly recently and he was completely on his own. The meals in the orphanage were served at long refectory tables with the children sitting on long benches. He had accidentally spilled a mug of cocoa and was taken by one of the nuns around the tables, in front of all the other children, to see the administrator who sat on a chair at the top of a pulpit where she could watch the children eating. He imagined he would be sent down to hell and was overwhelmed with terror.

We can now begin to see a connection between a current event, unresolved feelings from the past, and this father's irrational behaviour and depression. His anger and irritation with his daughter had nothing to do with her spilling the drink in the present, but everything to do with what was happening in his life when he spilled a drink when he was a small child. The tension he had felt, followed by the depression, were displaced emotions from his infancy.

The mechanism of displacement, as a defence against aggression, is fairly universal amongst children. They are physically weaker, more vulnerable and more dependent than adults. Behaving in an aggressive manner, particularly when the person you are angry with is also someone on whom you are dependent for your well-being, is risky. The more uncertain the relationship, the greater the risk and the more likely that hostile impulses will be displaced away from the source of hostility. On the other hand, if the relationship (with the parents or carers) is strong, if the child has experience of his or her anger being contained and thought about, then the need to deny or get rid of destructive impulses, by whatever method – splitting, denial, repression or displacement – is lessened.

In trying to understand the reasons for aggressive behaviour, it is useful to have some idea of the kind of situations in which children are likely to feel or behave aggressively. I have already mentioned frustration, particularly of instinctual needs (food, warmth, stimulation, nurturing), fear (of threats to the self or attachment figures) and loss of love. These are, of course, not exclusive categories. In reality, they are causally related and interact with each other at different levels. You cannot withdraw love from a child without inducing fear and, at some point, anger and aggression. On the other hand, if a child experiences too intense a frustration with his parent(s), he will react with anger and the anger will be experienced – in fantasy – as an attack on the good and caring relationship that he has with his parent(s) and a threat to the love that he has for them.

Other situations which frequently lead to aggression in children are: loss of containment (the capacity to 'hold' the child in one's mind both mentally and emotionally); being misunderstood; not feeling accepted; loss of self-esteem (ridiculing, teasing, denigrating or undervaluing the child); loss of control (this can happen when the structures which ensure that the child's world is safe, constant, predictable and reassuring are threatened, or when the child's own methods of coping fail); times of great stress or trauma and, finally, when there is a lowering of vitality due to illness or bereavement.

In addition to the foregoing, there are phases of development when there is a dramatic increase in the likelihood of childhood aggression. The most important of these occur around the age of two and prior to and during adolescence. Both of these phases are characterised by what may be described as fundamental changes in the child's relationship to his parents, to the outside world, and to himself.

### The 'terrible twos'

It is not without significance that the period between two and three years of age has been labelled by countless generations of parents as the 'terrible twos'. Children of this age can be extremely difficult, posing all kinds of problems for their parents especially in the testing out of boundaries and in their defiance, temper tantrums and omnipotent behaviour. If we examine all of the changes that are occurring at around this time – both internally and externally – I think we may be able to provide an explanation for something which has puzzled and sorely tried many parents and nursery teachers over the years.

The development of the child's awareness of himself as being both distinct and separate from his mother while relating in an intimate and intense way to her, probably evolves in the following manner. Initially, there is in all likelihood no differentiation between mother and child. Physically, mentally and emotionally, they are one. 'Magical thinking' (omnipotent hallucinatory gratification) is the order of the day. Almost before the sensations of hunger and discomfort or the need to be held and comforted can turn into emotions which would need to be thought about, they are satisfied by the mother who, if she is sufficiently identified or empathic with the baby, anticipates its needs before it becomes fully aware of them. This means that early on (in the first few months of life) the baby experiences very little disruption to the psychic state of undifferentiated at-oneness with the mother. Until it experiences frustration (of its instinctual needs) there is no sense of another. We do not have words in our lexicon to describe adequately this state of undifferentiatedness, of primary unity with the mother. The closest description to this state is probably the Sanskrit phrase used to describe nirvana (liberation) or samadhi (non attachment and non differentiation) *Sat-Chit-Ananda*: 'Being-Consciousness-Bliss'.

Unfortunately for the infant (but fortunately from the point of view of development and reality testing), external reality and instinctual needs have a habit of intruding into this blissful state and demanding that the baby acknowledges both the independent existence of the mother and his or her dependency upon her. In normal circumstances, this fundamental change in awareness comes about gradually, almost imperceptibly. By the time the baby realises that he and mother are not one; that *he* does not bring food, warmth, love, attention to himself merely through wishing for them (omnipotent hallucinatory gratification); that he is totally and absolutely dependent on her for everything; that he could not survive without her; it is also clear that his mother intuits his wishes and needs for him, that she willingly places his needs before hers. In this situation, although he loses his mother as a part of himself which he omnipotently controls, he finds her as someone separate, who *chooses* to be in relationship to him and who unselfishly gives him the love and understanding he needs. It is as though he goes from being the centre of his own universe, or more accurately, from being in a state of undifferentiated union with his mother (flowing over at-oneness), to him relating to her as a dependant satellite (but one which nourishes and feeds him), to the realisation that he is a dependant satellite that revolves around his mother who is at the centre of his universe/existence.

This realisation of his mother's autonomy and independence can be tolerated and accepted so long as she continues to gratify his needs and wishes. As soon as she shows a 'true' independence, where he has to accept and acknowledge that she has needs too, and where sometimes her needs and wishes take precedence over his, he begins to try to regain control over her and bend her to his will. At the same time, she is beginning to make demands on him. He cannot feed whenever he wants to, or demand her attention. There are *other people* with demands on her time that he has not really noticed until now.

Increasingly, he may have to take second place to father – or mother's partner – or even worse, another baby. All of this can lead to great unhappiness, misery, frustration and rage. This is made all the worse because by the time they have reached two years of age, most children are able to stand up and walk and manipulate their environment in a way which could not even be thought about before. Just being able to stand up enormously increases their range of vision and awareness of what is around them. However, it also brings home to them how little they can do compared to these giant-like figures who seem to know so much and who are so immensely powerful and competent. For some children, the realisation of their parents' awesome power and knowledge, allied to their awareness of their own limitations and dependency, is too much to bear. It is a tremendous blow to their self-love, self-esteem and sense of importance and they often retaliate or protest by being difficult, disobedient, spiteful and sometimes plain hateful.

## Aggression in adolescence

The next developmental phase where there is aggression in abundance, comes just prior to and during adolescence. There are several factors which make adolescence a fraught and trying time for all. The most obvious of these relates to physical changes in his or her external appearance and accompanying emotional and psychological changes that take place *within* the adolescent. These changes are sometimes very rapid and startling. A boy or girl can grow several inches in a few months. The girl will develop breasts, more rounded contours and begin to menstruate; the boy will develop a more muscular frame, a deeper voice and facial hair. In addition to acquiring secondary sexual characteristics, intense mood swings may be brought about by the impact of male and female 'sex hormones' which exert a powerful impact on the endocrine system. In both sexes, this can, and does, lead to an increase in irritability and aggressiveness.

Another factor which frequently leads to aggression and sometimes physical violence relates to changes in adolescents' relationships to their parents. The adolescent girl is now a young woman, and the adolescent boy, a young man. Both may now be as big or bigger than their parents. When they were younger, they took their parents as models and identified with them. Now they measure up to and challenge their parents. From copying their parents and idealising them, they begin to question and frequently to reject their earlier parental imagos. Part of this is healthy and normal. The earlier idealisation of the parents *needs* to be challenged by a less subjective and more objective view of them. You could say that, psychologically, children 'create the parents they need', and eventually, 'find the parents they have got.' Unfortunately, they are often disappointed and feel let down when they are mature enough to be able to see their parents in a more dispassionate light. This frequently leads to disillusion and a turning away from their parents' – and society's – values and belief systems. The less that adolescents can hold on to and continue to respect the internalised ideals of their parents, the more they are likely to look for alternative sets of values and belief systems, not necessarily because they believe in them, but because they contradict and oppose those of their parents.

Adolescence is, *par excellence*, a time of uncertainty, confusion, anxiety, excitement, challenge, misunderstanding and transformation. The leisurely meandering stream that could delight in the clear, sparkling water under blue skies and canopied trees is now a reckless, plunging, wild, out-of-control monster careering through dangerous rapids. The mature calm of deeper water and smoother passage has yet to come.

Perhaps the theme of 'transformation' is the key to understanding the enormous changes and resulting stresses and strains that accompany adolescence. Apart from the physical changes already referred to and the resulting changes in body image, there are psychological and social transformations which last throughout adolescence and frequently extend many years beyond it into adult life. The most difficult and profound of these relate to the changes which occur in the relationship between the adolescent and his or her parents. It is of course absolutely appropriate and in line with normal development that the adolescent boy or girl begins increasingly to look to his or her peers for support, self-affirmation, contact, friendship, love and affection, as well as role models. However, at the same time, he or she is losing his/her parents as a safe haven, as a major source of security and constancy, and has to face up to the challenges of sexual relations, the adult world, deciding on a career or getting a job. Increasingly, there are major events or challenges which they have to confront on their own and which their parents cannot, or should not, manage for them. *How* they manage them depends on the grounding they received from their parents. If this has been solidly established and adequate, then the adolescent can 'take off' from a secure base, confident both in his/her own abilities and qualities and in the ongoing love and support from parents. If not, then adolescence can be a painful, frightening, confusing and tormenting time.

For most of us, adolescence is a time of great ambivalence. The 'outside world' with all its mysteries, promises and enticements beckons with one hand, while the other finds it difficult to let go of the safety, security, comfort and protection of the family. Ideally, the letting go that must happen, occurs incrementally, in small steps, over an extended period of time. However, if the relationship with the parents has not been satisfactory, rather than this being a gradual process in which ongoing contact and good relations with parents is maintained it can be sudden, disruptive and violent. For many adolescents the only effective way to break with parents and achieve independence is by 'attacking' their parents and rejecting and denigrating everything they have stood for. If the parents respond in a hostile and rejecting way in return, this is then seen as a validation of the adolescent's aggressive and destructive behaviour and confirmation of their negative and sometimes denigratory view of their parents. In some ways, it is easier to achieve independence if you can maintain a negative, critical attitude towards your parents because then you have less to lose when you reject them.

## The communication of aggression

Aggression can be direct or indirect, covert or overt, owned or disowned. Aggression which is overt or direct is easier to recognise and, psychologically, easier to deal with. Physical assault, verbal abuse, defiance and attacks on property fall into this category. You may not understand why a child is aggressive, or what has caused it, but there is no mistaking the fact that it exists or how it is manifesting. Indirect or covert aggression is both harder to detect and much harder to deal with.

As mentioned above, in infancy aggressive feelings are experienced in relation to the primary object – namely, the mother – and that part of the self which is identified with the mother. Babies of course do show aggression; it is how they communicate when they are angry or distressed. Problems arise either when the anger is too intense and overwhelming or when the 'object' (mother/father) is not capable of containing or processing it and thus making it safe. When either of these are the case then the anger or aggression has to be denied and displaced. Typically, it is denied by the mechanisms of splitting and displacement, repression, or sublimation.

Before a functional ego is established, aggression which cannot be owned is split off, displaced, and projected into an object or person who, hopefully, is not harmed or destroyed by the aggressive impulses. Although the hostile impulses which are projected into, for instance, the mother, are not 'real' in the sense that they are omnipotent hallucinatory phantasies, the impact they have on the mother, both emotionally and psychologically, is real. Thus, the feelings evoked in the mother by her baby or infant can alert her to aggression which the baby may be experiencing but cannot communicate more directly, or which the baby or small child cannot afford to know about. The mother in this sense is acting as a 'transitional ego' which has the capacity to deal with the aggressive impulses of the child in a way in which the child cannot yet do. This means that the capacity to notice, observe, think about and process one's own internal reactions to children is essential if one is to be able to recognise and deal with aggression that has been subjected to the primitive mechanisms of splitting and projection.

When anger or aggression is repressed, rather than split off and projected, it may become turned in on the self. This can happen in several ways. The most primitive of these is via *somatisation*. Very early on in development, the mind and body are not clearly differentiated from the other either psychically or experientially. Sensations, feelings, and emotions are the prototypes for consciousness and for mental processes in general and they remain connected and to some extent interconnected to the extent that one can influence the other and, at times, *act as a substitute for the other*. When a hostile thought or emotion cannot be safely projected into a parent, or dissipated in any other way, then it may be transformed (by way of the genetic link between sensations and thinking) into something physical. 'Psycho-somatic' – 'Mind-Body' – implies exactly this, a causal connection between the two.

There are several illnesses – both physical and psychological – in which one of the factors in their aetiology is probably aggression which has had to be repressed. These are: asthma, eczema, migraine, anorexia nervosa, bulimia, encopresis and enuresis. In addition, there are several types of self-harm or masochistic behaviours which probably have a similar aetiology including: cutting and mutilation, drug or alcohol dependency, and head-banging.

I have shown how diverse and difficult to detect some forms of aggression are. What I would now like to look at are different ways of intervening with aggression and at the general principles underlying these interventions.

## Interventions and strategies for dealing with aggression: basic guidelines

The most important asset any of us has for dealing with aggression – whether in other people or ourselves – is situated on top of our shoulders: our brains. If we used it properly, then much of the aggression we see around us would be minimised or dealt with more effectively. The problem is that aggression is capable of stirring up primitive feelings and responses which tend to overcome or cloud our judgement and our capacity to think clearly and strategically. In some situations, it is appropriate to react automatically and without too much thought because time is of the essence. If someone is going to punch you on the nose, don't intellectualise, 'duck'! However, there are situations where being proactive instead of reactive can be a very effective way of dealing with aggression. With recurring or predictable scenarios where aggression is likely, you can sometimes pre-empt it, either by behaving in a way that would diminish the likelihood of an aggressive situation developing, or by responding at its onset in a way that *does not fit in with the expectations of the child*.

The following guidelines are only tentative. Rules are not made to be broken, but neither should they be followed as if they were written on tablets of stone. It is the interaction between rules and one's experience and intuition which makes them effective, not dogmatic adherence.

*Overt aggression*

In my opinion, the most important principle for managing aggression is containment. This can be physical, psychological, or a combination of both. When a baby behaves in an aggressive way towards its mother and she responds by holding it, speaking softly to it and trying to find out what is troubling it, she is 'containing' its anxiety and hostility. The baby's experience of being held and understood rather than punished or rejected, when repeated over time, helps it to tolerate situations in which aggression is a likely outcome. Containment also acts internally on the mother in that if she understands the reason for her child's aggression and its impact on her then she can better contain her own emotional responses rather than just be taken over by them.

Containment can also be provided by the environment. With the infant, the mother *is* the environment. With the older child, the setting of clear boundaries, rules and sanctions can be very effective in helping the child to contain his/her aggressive impulses. This is important because later in life, when parents are no longer there to 'lay down the law', the child who has been provided with parental containment as well as the containment provided by knowledge of the consequences of aggression, will have internalised both the way his parents dealt with aggression (their own and his) and the rules and prohibitions associated with it.

As I have already suggested, whenever possible, one should try to respond to aggression proactively rather than reactively. This may sound as though I am saying that you should never respond in a spontaneous or intuitive way. I am not. However, with repeated practice, it is possible to 'react proactively' in the sense that you can come up with a strategic response almost without thinking, just as, once you have mastered the techniques for driving a car, you no longer have to think them through. They become automatic.

Particularly when you are dealing with children who have a low threshold for frustration, the use of strategies and paradoxical injunctions can be very effective in containing, deflecting or defusing aggressive situations.

*Strategies and paradoxical injunctions*

Strategies are planned responses to a situation. They set out to 'change the rules' which the individual uses to make sense of, and regulate, both his behaviour and the way he relates to other people. Their effectiveness lies in the way in which they challenge the implicit assumptions and expectations the child has concerning the operation of 'rules of behaviour'. Because they go against the child's expectations, do not conform to the normal rules of logic and are not explained, they are difficult to circumvent by the child. Strategies which confound logic in this way are called paradoxical injunctions and their use in therapy has been employed in the main by family therapists, particularly Palazzoli, Milton Erickson, Carl Whitaker and Jay Haley.

Let me give you some examples of the thinking behind, and the operation of, strategic interventions in dealing with aggression in children.

A girl of ten in foster care was in danger of being rejected by the foster parents because of her unacceptably aggressive behaviour towards her foster mother whom she would verbally abuse and physically attack. The intervention I suggested was a paradoxical one. I said that the next time she was attacked she should immediately attack her husband in a similar manner. She should not say anything which would be unacceptable to him nor harm him physically but she must act as though she meant it. She also had to get her husband's agreement and co-operation as it was essential they work together as a team. Her husband, who was present at the consultation, was very taken aback by what I proposed but agreed to give it a go. His wife (as you might expect!) was rather taken by what was suggested and found it very amusing.

At the follow-up consultation, the foster mother told me that she and her husband had tried out the strategy. The next time her foster daughter began to behave aggressively towards her, she had turned on her husband and given him a tongue lashing. The reaction of her foster daughter was initially one of surprise, quickly followed by concern for the foster father. She had actually stepped in between them to protect him from his wife's anger. The immediate result of the strategy was that the girl stopped abusing her foster mother. Its effectiveness can be put down to the fact that the foster mother *took control of the symptom*. The symptom was aggression and *she* became the one who had the aggression. The fact that it was play-acted aggression only served to add to the confusion and disorientation provoked, firstly by the foster mother's aggression (she reversed role, going from helpless victim to controlling aggressor), and secondly, because the foster parents acted afterwards as if nothing had happened. In systemic terms, they challenged the rules and the expectations that the girl had, certainly implicitly, regarding her aggressive behaviour. Finally, her foster parents' behaviour provided her with an alternative model for dealing with aggression – one where aggression could be tolerated, manipulated and contained.

In my second example, an adolescent girl was behaving in such a contemptuous, denigrating and verbally aggressive manner towards her father that his wife feared he would suffer a heart-attack because of the stress it was causing him. The strategy proposed involved the wife taking control over the abusing situation. I suggested that she should take the initiative away from her daughter by pre-empting the abuse. Every time she sensed the daughter's aggression, she was to abuse her husband Once again, this was planned with the full co-operation and agreement of both parties to the strategy.

The first occasion to use the strategy arose during an evening meal. As soon as the daughter began to wind up to attacking her father, the mother pushed back her chair, picked up her husband's glass of wine and calmly poured it over his head. She then carried on eating and talking to her husband as though nothing unusual had happened. When I asked them how their daughter had reacted they both burst out laughing because the look of shock, disbelief and confusion that came over her had been so comical. Her husband had also been surprised but quickly recovered his internal composure when he realised that his wife was using the strategy they had both agreed upon. Using this kind of shock tactic, they completely undermined the abusive behaviour of their daughter. After all, what could *she* do that was worse than what her mother was doing?

Once again, the important factor in managing the aggression was to take control of it. Secondly, from the daughter's point of view, she saw her father being treated in the most appalling way and not being affected by it. His newly found imperviousness to aggression undermined whatever reward or gratification she obtained by attacking him. Thirdly, it joined them together as a couple and prevented her from causing splits between them. Finally, it dramatically reduced the tension, unhappiness and sense of impotence which the parents had been experiencing. *It empowered them.* This was made quite clear when they fed back in a following consultation. They both had tears in their eyes from laughing as they recounted the amazed disbelief in their daughter's face as her father continued eating his meal, with wine dripping from his hair onto his plate, and calmly asked his wife if she wouldn't mind filling up his glass again.

Not all strategies have to involve wasting good wine or pretending to lose your temper with someone. The important element is that whatever strategy is decided upon, it must be focused and directed at the perceived source of the problem or difficulty. It should be based on an understanding of the personalities, relationships and motivations of the people involved; it must be a strategy which is acceptable to those involved in putting it into action and it must *never* be explained to the person(s) it is directed at. Its main impact and effectiveness comes from the element of surprise. Its aim is to unbalance, to disorientate, to shock. These principles are essentially the same as those practised to such good effect by the Special Air Service (SAS): to confuse, disorientate and take control of a situation.

Although it is not literally a battle, and one should not even think of using strategic interventions to attack or harm one's children, it is useful, metaphorically speaking, to think of the aggressive child as an 'opponent' who has to be outmanoeuvred. If you *were* going into battle, you would certainly want to find out as much as you could about the enemy's disposition, their strengths and weaknesses, the location of their supply routes, reinforcements, the geography of the terrain and about their strategies and tactics in past encounters. Once you had this information, you would formulate a plan, a strategy, and prepare alternate strategies as back-ups in case the original one failed in its objective. You most certainly would not let the enemy know in advance, either what you had found out about them or what your intentions were.

It is always important – where you can – to keep a cool head. If your thinking gets contaminated by aggression or fear it always makes the situation worse (You can use aggression or simulate rage or fear if it is part of a strategy – then it is under your control). Team work is essential. A child who can split the adults responsible for its care can then play them off one against the other. For example, if one parent says 'No, you cannot have another biscuit', and the other says 'Yes', you may as well give up and give the child the biscuit tin! Be fair and be reasonable. On occasions, it is *very* difficult not to retaliate and be as nasty, vicious, persecuting and unreasonable as the child is. Don't. It isn't worth it. It will just make things worse. Besides, when a child is behaving in an unreasonable and unfair way, he *knows*. He may not acknowledge it at the time, but if you are fair and straight with him, he may acknowledge it later on. At any rate, whether he does or does not, he will respect you for it. Giving an aggressive child space and some room for manoeuvre (not too much), can help avoid explosive situations. Allied to taking control of the symptom, this can be very effective in containing and defusing hostile situations.

If a child, for example, is habitually unable to contain his/her aggression, then coming down on them too hard, giving them no room for manoeuvre, may escalate the situation. Saying things like, 'I am going to give you ten minutes/half an hour to think about it, then such and such will happen' is far better than saying, 'Stop it now or else!' Another useful tactic is to find a shared nick-name for the aggressive or 'naughty' part of the child, and then to address the child by their 'normal' name in an attempt to forge a 'benign split' between the part of the child that can be thoughtful, responsive and in control, and the part that cannot. With one very aggressive child, I suggested to his parents that they ask him what name he would give to the angry part of himself. After thinking about it for a while, he decided to call it 'Lurch'. They were then to tell him to take 'Lurch' up to his room whenever Lurch had misbehaved and keep him there until he had calmed down. The father told me that when he told his son to take 'Lurch' to his room when he had been threatening his brother, he went up to his room without the usual protest. When he did not come down again, the father went to find out what was happening. His son told him that he could not come down yet because 'Lurch was still angry and he was going to keep him there until he had calmed down'. Creating a 'benign split' between the aggressive part of the child's personality and the part which could relate to it in an objective and thoughtful way allowed this boy to have more control over his aggressive impulses. You could say that it helped him to develop a 'witnessing' part of his ego where one part could witness or observe the functioning of another part and thereby better understand and control it.

## Unconscious or hidden aggression

As I have already indicated, indirect or covert aggression is harder to detect and to deal with than overt aggression. In the infant or small child this is because:

1. In fantasy (both conscious and unconscious), aggression directed towards the loved object is experienced as equivalent to the deed. This is due to the fact that the infant cannot differentiate between fantasy and reality. The thought *is* the deed. Therefore the primitive mechanisms of splitting and projection are mobilised to ensure that, where possible, hostile impulses are detached and located away from the self.

2. If you as the parent or caretaker are the recipient of these projected impulses, it is not always apparent whose feelings belong to whom.

With the older child who is more able to discriminate between fantasy and reality, and between self and other, the range of defences available to deny, distort or hide aggressive impulses is much greater. They can be subject to inversion or reaction formation in which impulses are changed into the opposite. For example, the wish to get rid of, hurt or murder a baby brother or sister who has come along to replace you in mother's or father's affections can be disguised by exaggerated displays of affection. Sometimes, in spite of the 'best' of intentions, baby gets dropped, hit, knocked over, hugged too hard or stuffed with food to the point of choking.

Another sign of hidden aggression is associated with frequent 'accidents' in which either another child gets hurt or valued items of furniture or personal possessions keep getting damaged. If one begins to observe a pattern to these incidents, it may become possible to address the underlying motive of hostility in a more conscious way in which it can be spoken about. The adopted son of a schoolteacher, who was afraid that if he showed any aggression he would be placed back into care, had been damaging items of her clothing or valued pieces of furniture in such a way that she could never be sure that he was responsible. He had, for example, pulled out single strands of thread from a favourite dress and made hairline scratches on the highly polished surface of a dressing table. He had probably been doing this for months before she was convinced that all of these 'accidents' were in fact intentional.

In therapy, I was able to discover that the true focus of his hostility was directed at his biological parents who had never been able to care for him properly. When he was with them, any display of emotion was severely punished. Early on in therapy he painted a large red heart underneath which he had written 'TRUE LOVE...'. On the opposite page he painted another large red heart but this time with black cracks zigzagging across it. It was a heart – his heart – which had been broken and was in pieces. Underneath this heart he wrote '...NEVER LASTS'. On one level, he had displaced his anger and hostility from his rejecting parents onto his adoptive mother. On the other, he was terribly afraid that if he showed it, he would be rejected once again. However, he needed to know if his adoptive mother could survive his hostility. Without knowing this, he would never feel secure. Fortunately, she was very attached to him and the understanding he gained in therapy meant that he no longer felt the need to disguise or hide his anger in the same manner.

In dealing with aggression in children and learning how to manage and respond to it, it is important to understand that no matter how extreme or unreasonable it is, it *is* a communication and, although it may have to be reacted to – sometimes with one's own aggression – it should always be thought about and an attempt made to understand it. The very fact that one takes as given that aggression has meaning, function and purpose *beyond the physical fact of violence* helps one to hold back from over-reacting and getting emotionally caught up by the aggression being displayed. If you can contain, think about and process what is happening – inside the child as well as inside yourself – that is the first step in helping the child manage, make sense of and find alternative ways of dealing with the causes of aggression.

## References

Bowlby, J. (1972) *Attachment.* Harmondsworth: Pelican Books.

Frankl, V.E. (1969) *Man's Search For Meaning.* New York: Washington Square Press.

Lorenz, K. (1970) *On Aggression.* London: Methuen and Co. Ltd.

Mahler, M.S., Pine, F. and Bergman, A. (1987) *The Psychological Birth of the Human Infant.* London: Maresfield Library.

Tustin, F. (1981) *Autistic States in Children.* London: Routledge and Kegan Paul.

Winnicott, D.W. (1976) *The Maturational Processes and the Facilitating Environment.* London: Hogarth Press and the Institute of Psycho-Analysis.

# CHAPTER 6

# Troubles of Sexuality

*Francis Dale*

In humans, sexuality can be defined as, *a biological urge or instinct which passes through several developmental stages – physiological, emotional, psychological and cultural – usually with the ultimate aim of establishing the sexual union of the mature male and female for the purpose of procreation.* In the vast majority of cultures, the context of the end purpose of adult sexuality – giving birth to and raising children – is the nuclear or extended family, composed of mother, father and related kin.

Because of the long period of dependency on parents, the profound influence of 'learned patterns of behaviour', the threat to the nuclear family from divorce and breakdown, and the increasing impact of cultural influences from outside the immediate family, the normal development of 'healthy' patterns of sexual behaviour is becoming more and more difficult to achieve. However, before we can begin to be able to understand deviant or pathological sexuality, we need to have some notion of, and clarity concerning, normal sexual development.

Although it was published at the turn of the century and has generated much debate and controversy Freud's *Three Essays on the Theory of Sexuality* is still one of the seminal and most profound pieces of writing on the psychological nature of sexuality and its roots in infancy. He introduced various terms and concepts, including 'libido', to describe the force or the energy of the sexual instinct; the various developmental stages through which the infant's sexuality manifests and progresses – oral, anal and genital; and the notion that sexuality in the infant is *polymorphously perverse.* Freud believed that the earliest impulses of sexuality in the infant could be attributed to a combination of sensuous excitation in the various erogenous zones and the satisfaction of the vital functions necessary for survival. The mouth, for example, is an organ for the taking in of nourishment while at the same time the act of sucking can induce the most intense states of blissful sensuality and sexual excitation. As an illustration of the connection between sucking (in this case thumb-sucking) and sexual pleasure, Freud quotes the following description of a young woman in his *Three Essays on the Theory of Sexuality*:

> Not every kiss is equal to a 'Lutscherli' [i.e. sucking one's thumb] – no, no not by any means! It is impossible to describe what a lovely feeling goes through your whole body when you suck; you are right away from this world. You are absolutely satisfied and happy beyond desire. It is a wonderful feeling; you long for nothing but peace – uninterrupted peace. It is just unspeakably lovely: you feel no pain and no sorrow, and ah! You are carried into another world. (Freud 1986, p.181)

He sees, in the infant's early relationship to the breast and the feeding mother, a prototype of adult sexual fulfilment:

> No one who has seen a baby sinking back satiated from the breast and falling asleep with flushed cheeks and a blissful smile can escape the reflection that this picture persists as a prototype of the expression of sexual satisfaction in later life. (p.182)

Freud is clearly implying an underlying connection between the infant's blissful, sensual satisfaction centred around the function of feeding and the genital satisfaction of later sexual relationships: '…the first impulses of sexuality make their appearance attached to other vital functions… [W]hen children fall asleep after being sated at the breast, they show an expression of blissful satisfaction which will be repeated later in life after the experience of sexual orgasm.' (Freud 1974, p.355).

The implications of the connection between the infant's sensual nurturing relationship to the mother and the development of sexual behaviour and attitudes are of considerable importance in understanding various problems which can arise relating to sexuality. This is because the roots of our sexuality are laid down and consolidated in the first few months of life in that extraordinarily intimate relationship to the nurturing mother.

## Sexuality in infancy

### The oral stage

Although we cannot really know for certain what a baby thinks about (or even if it can 'think' at all given the lack of neuronal myelination and cortical development), we can, through observation and inference, draw some tentative conclusions regarding its probable early experience. To begin with, it is highly unlikely that the neonate has any conscious awareness of itself as 'self' or of the mother as 'other'. It is probably in a state of 'primary undifferentiated at-oneness' with the mother – which we might describe as 'being, conscious-ness, bliss'. Margaret Mahler describes this as a phase of normal symbiosis, 'in which the infant behaves and functions as though he and his mother were an omnipotent system – a dual unity within one common boundary…[a] state of undifferentiation, of fusion with the mother, in which the "I" is not yet differentiated from the "not I" and in which inside and outside are only gradually coming to be sensed as different' (Mahler, Pine and Bergman 1987, p.44).

Thus when the baby is feeding from the breast, it is *psychically* feeding from the breast *as self.* That is to say, to begin with, all pleasurable and unpleasurable experiences are subjective and intrapsychic. We can observe this with very young babies when they are feeding. Many mothers have noticed how what seems to them an insignificant event can have a profound and long-lasting impact on their babies. The kind of thing I am thinking about is how disturbing an intrusion is to the suckling infant. A sudden noise, a cough, a sneeze, the telephone ringing, and the infant frequently reacts, first with a startled response, and then with acute signs of disturbance. It is as if the intrusion threatens the primary undifferentiated unity with the maternal object, the breast. One has the impression that the mouth–nipple contact in some way 'holds the baby together' and at the same time provides the baby with sensual gratification of a most blissful kind. What we have here is a phenomenon which Freud remarked on in the *Three Essays* – namely, that an activity which satisfies the infant's need for nourishment also has an erotic component. Not only that, but an erotic component which makes itself *independent* of the instinctual urge for nourishment. Many auto-erotic behaviours bear no relationship to feeding but seem to be indulged in purely for the degree of pleasure they give to the baby.

If we consider the fact that at birth there are as many sensory nerve endings in the skin as in maturity, then, given the much smaller surface area of skin in the baby, we can assume that the skin of the baby is, correspondingly, much more sensitive and responsive to touch and innervations. That is to say, the skin of the baby is capable of providing significantly more pleasurable sensations than that of the adult. We know that touching and stroking the skin – even in areas that are not directly connected to the sexual organs – can enhance sexual pleasure in adults. It would be hard to deny then, that stroking the skin of the baby provides a similar kind of intense pleasure that, later on in development, becomes associated with and integral to, genital sexuality. Freud defined sexual activity as perverse if it did not have the aim of reproduction as its end result and pursued the attainment of pleasure independently from it (Freud 1974, p.358). Given that it is many years before children – let alone babies – are capable of full genitality and reproduction, we should not refer to sexual behaviour in infants and small children as perverse but more as infantile sexuality in which the stimulation of organs not specifically designated as sexual, nor yet functioning in a sexual way, can provoke an orgasmic type of pleasure.

If we turn now from the skin as an organ, the stimulation of which can provide intense sensual pleasure, to a highly specialised part of it responsible for ingestion – the mouth and lips – we can, as with the skin in general, assume that it too is highly sensitised and capable of providing the baby with highly pleasurable sensations. That these sensations become associated with and part of genital sexuality there can be no doubt but they are rooted in infantile sexuality. As Freud so appositely puts it:

> If an infant could speak, he would no doubt pronounce the act of sucking at his mother's breast by far the most important in his life. He is not far wrong in this, for in this single act he is satisfying two great vital needs. We are therefore not surprised to learn from psychoanalysis how much psychical importance the act retains all through life. Sucking at the mother's breast is the starting point of the whole of sexual life, the unmatched prototype of every later sexual satisfaction, to which phantasy often recurs in time of need. This sucking involves making the mother's breast the first object of the sexual instinct. (Freud 1974, p.356)

The mother is, therefore, the infant's first love object and as the love the baby has for the mother, particularly in its sensual aspect, lays the foundation for later sexual attitudes and predispositions, any problems in the way the infant and mother relate to each other at this stage can have lasting consequences on the direction and outcome of adult sexual behaviour.

### Problems in the relationship between mother and child

It is only at the point at which the infant becomes aware of the separate existence – at first purely physical – of himself and his mother that we can begin to talk of a relationship, in any objective sense of the word, between mother and child. Once there is a dyad, as opposed to an undifferentiated at-oneness, power, control, and projections of both a positive and negative nature become operative in both directions. The baby has to feel secure in the knowledge that his basic needs will be met. Initially this happened automatically – almost magically – without thought or much effort on his part. His wishes and their automatic satisfaction led to a belief or an expectation in omnipotent hallucinatory gratification. Now, someone else's wishes have to be taken into account.

In the normal run of things, the mother's receptiveness (Winnicott's (1976) 'primary maternal preoccupation') ensures that she responds appropriately to the baby's primary needs. For some babies, however, in a way that is still not properly understood, the baby does not appear to be able to trust that the breast will be there for him unless he can control it in some way. There ensues what can only be called a 'battle for the breast'. Some babies do seem to be constitutionally more aggressive or assertive than other babies. Either way, it is a 'battle' which the mother must win – both for herself and for her baby. If she fails, she may end up having a baby who, when he is feeding, seems to take no account of *her* feelings or even to acknowledge her as a separate person. Her breasts belong to him and she is the servant, or worse, slave, who fulfils his every need. In this scenario, the baby's earlier omnipotence is not moderated and softened by coming up against the reality of his mother's separate existence and his dependence on her. The mother's failure – when appropriate developmentally – to stand up to her baby's omnipotence can be due to several different factors. One may be because the mother does not feel supported by the father or other male figures who do relate to her as a woman who is valued in her person and not just in her body. Another may be connected to her projecting *her* unmet infantile needs into her baby which she then, unconsciously, seeks to satisfy, even though, as a parent, she becomes the victim of her own infantile omnipotence (now projected into her baby).

Whatever the reason, if the baby's omnipotence in gratifying its narcissistic needs goes unchecked, there is a risk that later sexual development will produce an individual with marked narcissistic and sadistic trends whose sexuality is primarily expressed at the expense of other individuals who are related to solely in terms of meeting one's own needs. One might talk here about a 'greedy', 'gobbling up' kind of sexuality where the primary objective in relating to others is in terms of taking from, denuding and controlling rather than giving, sharing and reciprocating.

Some years ago a boy of six was referred to me because of severe behavioural problems both at home and at school. 'Martin' was very wilful, defiant and manipulative and was almost beyond control – only doing something or co-operating if it suited him. More worryingly, he could behave in a particularly sadistic way towards weaker more vulnerable children as well as female teachers who would often be reduced to tears by his cruel taunting and challenging behaviour. His parents had separated when he was just over a year old and he had been left with his mother who was unable to show any warmth towards him. When he was excluded from his first primary school his mother admitted that she could not cope with his destructive and aggressive behaviour and his father offered to look after him.

In therapy, he offered a striking picture. On the one hand, he could be very cold, calculating, denigrating, omnipotent and extremely manipulative; on the other, he would behave like a very small baby wanting me to look after him and to be controlled by him like a captive, servant mother. Disturbingly, I never felt that I mattered to him. I was only useful in as much as I *was* useful. I came to see that he had no notion, experience or interest in relating to other people in a mutually reciprocal way. He seemed to lack any conscience or morality. People were there to be used by him – either for his pleasure, or as receptacles to take his pain, hurt and frustration. He was one of the most destructive children (in the emotional sense of the word) that I have ever come across. He was an expert in eliciting hope in other people and then destroying and rubbishing it.

When he was ten he was again excluded from school and sent to a residential school for disturbed children where I continued to see him, more to provide some sense of continuity than in the hope that he could be reached by once weekly therapy. Eventually I had to stop seeing him because he behaved in ways which made it impossible to continue seeing him for analytical psycho-therapy in the setting in which he was being treated.

At the age of 16, he was charged with sexually abusing a young girl and offered further counselling. He showed no remorse, only concern at having been caught out. From my understanding of the disturbed relationship he had had with his mother, his inability to own any feelings of dependency or neediness in therapy, and the omnipotent and manipulative way in which he related to other people, I had thought it likely that something like this would happen when he reached adolescence and became sexually mature. For him, his sexuality was not part of a mature, integrated personality based on a satisfactory loving relationship with the breast but more a commodity and a means of satisfying his own urges regardless of the 'other'.

There is another kind of difficulty which relates more to the 'greediness of the breast'. This can have two sources. One relates to primitive phantasies stemming from the time when infant and breast were not differentiated from each other. Detailed observations of the feeding infant suggest that when the impulse to feed is too strong (this may be due to excessive frustration at delays in feeding) the devouring hunger the infant experiences is projected into the breast which then becomes related to as a *devouring breast*. Here, the infant's overwhelming greed is denied, split off and located in the mother where it can more easily be defended against. Alternatively, at an unconscious level, the mother may project into the baby her own infantile greed in which case there will be an objective reality to the infant's experience of the breast as devouring and intrusive. When older children, who have moved into the genital phase of sexual development, visualise the infantile fear of being taken over and gobbled up by the devouring 'mother/breast' they typically draw either a vagina with sharp teeth or sometimes a spider in a web.

The defences erected against the devouring breast or vagina can, if untreated, have an influence on later sexual attitudes. In the male child, one of these is homosexuality, particularly of a passive, compliant type. Another can be impotence: the fear of the potent phallus being that it can be 'swallowed up' by the devouring vagina. Yet another could be sexual sadism based on a desire for revenge against the terrifying female sexual imago. Here, the potency of the phallus is used as a 'weapon' to punish, damage, humiliate or control the terrifying female 'predator'.

An adult patient of mine had fantasies about doing damage to his partners in the act of sexual intercourse whilst at the same time suffering from impotence. They were both connected and could be traced back to anger towards his mother for abandoning him when he was a toddler and her using him to satisfy her sexual and emotional needs. In some ways this was very exciting for him and made him feel very close and special to her. It also filled him with disquiet, guilt and anxiety about being caught up and taken over by something which was beyond his control and understanding.

Due to the enormous significance of learning and individual differences on behaviour, it would be unwise as well as misleading to imply a causal one-to-one relationship between any particular aspect of the baby's feeding relationship and later sexual attitudes. One can, however, point to likely or probable outcomes, which is not the same as claiming scientific validity. Most of our understanding of the influences on our sexuality – particularly of the oral phase of development – are *post hoc* and based on inferences drawn from observation of babies and children and work with adults.

## The anal stage

The next phase of development introduces the infant, for perhaps the first time, to the necessity of controlling and suppressing a natural urge which also provides it with auto-erotic stimulation, namely, the act of defecation. Apart from weaning, which may not yet have taken place, this begins the long road to civilisation and conformity to the rules and prescriptions of those on whom one is dependent. It also introduces the infant to delayed gratification. It cannot defecate where and when it wishes to (this is not true of some primitive societies which we will discuss later (p.92)). According to both Freud (1974) and Abraham (1973) certain distinctive character traits in neurotic individuals are typically associated with what is called the 'anal character'. These are: an obsessive orderliness, meanness or acquisitiveness and defiant obstinacy. Because the mucosal membranes of the anus are richly endowed with sensory neurones, stimulation of it provides the child with pleasurable erotic feelings – either from the act of defecation, or from external manipulation.

As we have already seen, the pleasure associated with an instinct, such as suckling, can become detached from its original function and independent of it. In this way, the anus can become invested with great significance as the source of immense riches which are, in unconscious phantasy, felt to be located 'inside one's bottom'. In extreme situations of either under- or over-evaluation, the anus can become a substitute genital and the dominant focus for sexual excitation. Children who are understimulated or unloved will frequently turn, or regress to, auto-erotic activities such as thumb sucking or anal masturbation as a substitute for normal object relations (i.e. a healthier, mutually reciprocal way of relating to parent or significant other). If this state of affairs persists, the child may turn away from seeking gratification and pleasure in relationships in the normal way, fearing that in any relationship in which it has to give it will be depleted. In this manner, feelings or emotions tend to be hoarded and held on to and, by extension, other things, such as possessions, cannot easily be shared or given up.

Children who are over-valued frequently develop grandiose ideas concerning their self-importance which, if not counteracted by reality testing, can result in them turning into narcissistic individuals whose only interest is in themselves and their own personal gratification. They too cannot give as everything has to centre around their need to be the centre of attention and of other people's admiration and envy. Because during the anal phase of development the child is gaining control and power over his body and its functions, he is increasingly able to turn to himself to replace those gratifications for which previously he had to depend on the object (his mother) to fulfil. If the child can trust that his mother can respond to and satisfy his sensual and emotional needs, there is less likelihood of him turning away from object relating and attempting to meet those instinctual needs in a narcissistic, auto-erotic way. If not, then his later sexuality will not be about object relating – about giving and receiving intimacy – but about treating people as 'things' whose sole function is to provide him (or her) with sensual gratification, regardless of *their* needs. The move from 'self' to 'other' is paralleled in psychoanalytic thought by the move from anal to genital primacy. To quote from Karl Abraham:

> It is only by degrees that it [the child] overcomes to some extent its egoistic impulses and its narcissism and takes the step towards object love…this stage of development coincides with another important event, namely, attainment of the highest level of libidinal development – the genital level…the individual is able to fill his place and exercise his powers fully and satisfactorily in his social environment only if his libido has reached the genital stage… The first function of this third stage in the formation of character is…to get rid of the remaining traces of the more primitive stages of development, in so far as they are unfavourable to the social behaviour of the individual. For he will not, for instance, be able to achieve a tolerant and fair minded attitude to other people and to interests *outside his own* [my italics] until he has got the better of his destructive and hostile impulses springing from sadistic sources, or of his avarice and mistrust derived from oral ones. (Abraham 1973, p.408)

*The genital stage*

This is the final developmental stage (preceded by the oral and anal stages) which plays a significant, if not crucial, role in determining the direction and outcome of sexual development. It is immediately preceded by a phase of development called latency in which there appears to be a diminution of the previous interest and preoccupation in sexual explorations and activities. It is not that sexuality has ceased to be a pressing and urgent concern but that it has, as it were, 'gone underground' and become latent. There is general agreement that this is because the development of both a personal and social conscience imposes constraints and limitations on the immediate gratification of instinctual impulses via the agency of what is called the super ego. As mentioned above, impulses can increasingly be deferred, sublimated or suppressed in line with what is considered acceptable to the individual.

This gives the young adolescent time to incorporate, assimilate and integrate the vast amount of new experiences and learning tasks that are part of growing up and moving out into the world, and into extra-familial relationships, without being too overwhelmed by the intense emotional disturbances that are part of genital sexuality. At first, however, a major hurdle has to be overcome and this relates to what Freud called the Oedipus conflict. This takes its name from the Greek tragedy by Sophocles in which a child, Oedipus, who was abandoned and left for dead by his parents, returns as an adult and unknowingly kills his father and marries his mother. At around the age of three or four, both boys and girls are confronted with the reality that someone else has a 'special' and sexually exclusive relation with mother. This has the potential to stir up tremendous rage, envy, guilt, despair and rejection. From being a dyadic relationship it has now become a triangular relationship where father and mother share intimacies from which the child can feel excluded.

In the majority of cases, the situation is made more bearable by the fact that the child also has a loving and nurturing relationship with the father and, in particular, that the father becomes an important figure of attachment in his own right. The dilemma is resolved – and only ever partially – through various kinds of compromise formation:

> For the boy, [this] is primarily by identification with the father. In some ways the father is a more powerful, exciting and intriguing figure than the mother. The exclusive relationship to the mother can be to some extent compensated for by developing a similarly exclusive relationship with the father. After all, son and father are the same. They both have a 'willy' and one day the boy will be big and powerful like his dad. The son can identify with his father in ways which he cannot with his mother. In addition, in unconscious identification with the father, the son can

have the same intimacy with his mother that his father does. He too can become her 'husband', her protector, her 'little man'.

For the girl, the situation is different. She can identify with her mother. She is the same sex. In one sense, like the male child, she 'loses' mother in having to share her with daddy. In another sense, she keeps mummy by identifying with her and becoming her in a way that is not possible in the boy's case. In identification with the mother, the girl both 'keeps' her but also replaces her. As with the boy's desire to get rid of the father, this creates unconscious guilt, for the girl also needs and loves her mother.

With both sexes, the identification with the parent of the same sex, in the boy's case with the father in order to possess the mother, in the girl's case with the mother in order to identify with her, is the source of much anxiety. This is because, in both cases, the identification has the unconscious significance of having replaced, for the boy, the father in mother's affections, and for the girl, the mother in father's affections. (Dale 1993, p.22)

In general, I think it is true to say that the resolution of the Oedipus conflict is held to be central to the development of healthy sexual relationships in adult life: '…when the child has been able to subdue his Oedipus complex with all its constituents he has made the most important step towards overcoming his original narcissism and his hostile tendencies; and at the same time he has broken the power of the pleasure-principle to dominate the conduct of his life.' (Abraham 1975, p.409)

## Failure to work through the Oedipus complex

Although anthropological studies do not unequivocally support Freud's contention that the Oedipal situation is a universal phenomenon and its resolution one of the essential preconditions for the existence of civilised societies, they do suggest that even in the most primitive societies an incest taboo is central to the regulation of sexual relationships and kinship structures. In addition, while in some primitive societies great freedom and permissiveness is granted to even very small children in their sexual explorations and activities, at adolescence and full sexual maturity, prohibitions, rules and rituals concerning all aspects of sexual behaviour come into play. In his seminal work, *The Sexual Life of Savages* (1929), in which he studied the sexual behaviour of the Trobriand Islanders of the South Seas, the anthropologist, Bronislaw Malinowski, found that children knew all the essentials of adult sexual behaviour from a very early age:

...children hear of and witness much of the sexual life of their elders. Within the house, where the parents have no possibility of finding privacy, a child has opportunities of acquiring practical information concerning the sexual act...no special precautions are taken to prevent children from witnessing their parents' sexual enjoyment. (p.54)

The children initiate each other into the mysteries of sexual life in a directly practical manner at a very early age. A premature amorous existence begins among them long before they are able really to carry out the act of sex. (p.55)

However, Malinowski reported acts of full sexual intercourse in girls between the ages of six and eight, and boys between the ages of ten to twelve. The finding that is of some significance for the present discussion is that, contrary to what we might expect, the prevalence of sexual perversions or sexual deviancy amongst adult South Sea Islanders was almost negligible. There are several likely explanations for this. One is in accordance with Freud's assertion that many of the sexual ailments of modern society (in his day, nineteenth century middle class Viennese society) are the result of overly rigid moral prescriptions resulting in the suppression of natural instinctual sexual impulses. Amongst the children of the South Sea Islanders there were few if any sexual prohibitions: 'The infantile sexual act, or its substitute, is regarded as an innocent amusement. It is their play to *kayta* (to have intercourse).' (Malinowski 1929, p.56). However, in many technological societies, given the amount of sexual permissiveness that obtains, the suppression of sexual behaviour in children cannot provide a sufficient explanation for the sexual problems of children and adolescents.

If there is an explanation, I think it lies more with alterations in the structure and functioning of the basic family unit, as well as in more widespread changes in cultural traditions. There can be little doubt that industrialisation has had a profound influence on the way we live our lives and particularly on the stability of family life. In their fascinating and engaging book *Family and Kinship in East London* (1970) two sociologists, Michael Young and Peter Wilmott, studied working-class East End families in Bethnal Green in London before, during and after a long-established community was relocated and rehoused on a purpose-built estate. From living in an extended community where everyone knew everyone else and where doors were unlocked and generations of families lived in the same street, families became dispersed, insular and cut off from the free and easy access to each other that they had previously enjoyed. In many ways, the children had been as much rooted in and 'held' by the community as they were by their immediate family. Family problems, day to day difficulties, the tensions and upsets of adolescence and sexuality could all be shared and made more bearable through the wider participation of the individual child in the kinship network.

In much of western society, there has been a steady erosion of such extended family and community support. Family culture, mores, traditions and rituals concerning the progression and nurturing of the child as he or she passes through the various stages of development is giving way to mass culture and the lack of mores and traditions of the mass media. Increasingly, children are having to find their own way in response to the lack of a 'way' that can be imbibed from their parents.

Empirical research from psychoanalysis suggests that, at least in Western culture, the optimal conditions for 'normal' heterosexual development occur in families where there is a stable, long-term relationship between father and mother. This stable relationship provides a focus and a model in respect to which sexual experiences and behaviour can be experienced in relative safety. It allows for the Oedipal situation to be worked through without too much anxiety and for sexual development to proceed in relation to the maturation of the personality as a whole. As Abraham points out in his 1925 paper on character formation (see Abraham 1973), there is a close connection between character formation and the psycho-sexual development of the child. The most significant factor in the way in which the character of the child – and hence its sexual behaviour – develops is the nature of its object relationships in early infancy and the successful working through of the Oedipus complex.

## Perverse sexuality

According to the analytic model of sexual development, deviant or perverse sexuality has its roots in

1. failure in attachment in early object relations

2. failure to negotiate the various stages of libidinal development

3. failure to resolve the Oedipal situation

4. the absence of a stable parental relationship that can act as a template against which one's own sexuality can emerge and flourish

5. distorted or disturbed sexual functioning in the parent(s).

If we set aside the rather narrow psychoanalytic definition of perversion as 'any form of adult sexual behaviour in which heterosexual intercourse is not the preferred goal' (Rycroft 1972, p.116) we can allow for a broader and more inclusive definition of 'normal' sexuality which *includes* deviations from the above definition. Freud himself in his *Introductory Lectures on Psychoanalysis* warned against making too rigid a demarcation between normal and perverse sexuality:

> However infamous they may be, however sharply they may be contrasted with normal sexual activity, quiet consideration will show that some perverse trait or other is seldom absent from the sexual life of normal people. (Freud 1974, p.364)

He believed this to be the case because he saw normal sexual development developing from the polymorphous sexuality of the child which cannot have as its aim the procreation and parenting of children.

In conclusion, we can say that problems of sexuality in childhood have their roots, and their resolutions, in the nature of the child's relationship with his parents and his culture as he passes through the various stages of development. In the familial and cultural vacuum in which many of our children are brought up there is an absence of norms, values, traditions, boundaries and appropriate role models to help them develop responsive and responsible attitudes to both their own and others' sexuality. Because sexual experience is designed to be pleasurable, for many it becomes an end in itself rather than the means to an end which is the bringing together of two people, not just to have sex and give each other sexual pleasure, but to produce children and to provide a caring, loving environment in which they can grow and flourish and in turn, pass on to their children what they have been given by their parents.

> Sex is not a mere physiological transaction to the South Islander any more than it is to us; it implies love and love-making; it becomes the nucleus of such venerable institutions as marriage and the family; it pervades art and it produces its spells and magic. It dominates in fact almost every aspect of culture. Sex in its widest meaning…is rather a sociological and cultural force than a mere bodily relation of two individuals. (Malinowski 1929, xxiii)

## References

Abraham, K. (1973) 'Character-Formation on the Genital Level of the Libido.' In *Selected Papers on Psycho-Analysis*. London: Hogarth Press and the Institute of Psycho-Analysis.

Dale, F.M.J. (1993) 'Unconscious communication of hatred between parents and children.' In V. Varma (ed) *How and Why Children Hate*. London: Jessica Kingsley Publishers.

Freud, S. (1974) *Introductory Lectures on Psychoanalysis*. Harmondsworth: Penguin Books.

Freud, S. (1986) *Three Essays on the Theory of Sexuality*. In *The Standard Edition*. London: Hogarth Press and the Institute of Psycho-Analysis.

Mahler, M.S., Pine, F. and Bergman, A. (1987) *The Psychological Birth of the Human Infant*. London: Maresfield Library.

Malinowski, B. (1929) *The Sexual Life of Savages*. New York: Harcourt, Brace and World, Inc.

Rycroft, C. (1972) *A Critical Dictionary of Psychoanalysis*. Harmondsworth: Penguin Books.

Winnicott, D.W. (1976) *The Maturational Processes and the Facilitating Environment.* London: Hogarth Press and the Institute of Psycho-Analysis.

Young, M. and Wilmott, P. (1970) *Family and Kinship in East London.* Harmondsworth: Penguin Books.

# CHAPTER 7

# Troubles of Adolescence

*David Fontana*

Received wisdom has it that adolescence is a period of storm and stress. The adolescent, poised uneasily between the world of the child and that of the adult, is seen as going through a period of extreme psychological and social upheaval, rocked by the onslaught of hormonal changes on the one hand, and by rebellion against the values and judgements of the grown-up world on the other. But how accurate is this picture? Research suggests it may owe less to the experience of adolescents themselves than to the social myth-making of their elders and betters. Coleman (1994) implies a connection between this myth-making and the two sets of theories that have been most influential in shaping our thinking about the adolescent years, namely psychoanalytical theories and sociological theories. We can examine in turn the models of adolescence generated by each of these sets of theories, and then proceed to the various other relevant models that have attempted to explain what happens during the sometimes turbulent transition from childhood to adulthood.

## The psychoanalytical model

For Freud, adolescence marks the genital stage of psychosexual development, that is the stage when the sexual instinct is claimed to become centred upon its primary erogenous zone, the genitals, and to be directed towards members of the opposite sex as the prime focus of sexual desire. As with the other psychosexual stages, unless there is an orderly process of maturation at this point, the individual may remain fixated in infantile dependencies, with the consequence that he or she may be unable to develop a personality free from the major neuroses, and adjust fully to a mutually rewarding relationship with a partner.

The severing of dependency ties with parents is termed *disengagement* in Freudian theory (see e.g. Lerner 1987), and constitutes for Freudians one of the major developmental tasks of adolescence. During the disengagement process, many adolescents show *regression* to forms of behaviour (such as emotional outbursts, withdrawal, wilfulness, self-doubt, misdirected aggression aimlessness, over-enthusiams, and emotional dependencies transferred from parents to peers) more appropriate to earlier stages of development (Blos 1967). Often linked at this time to regression is *ambivalence* – fluctuations in mood and behaviour, emotional instability, illogicality, and abrupt mood and behavioural swings between rejection and acceptance of people and ideas. Both regression and ambivalence have their root cause in the emotional uncertainty with which the adolescent regards parents and authority in general, fluctuating as he or she does between feelings of love and dependency, and of hatred and the desire for independence.

In addition to regression and ambivalence, Freudians see many of the difficulties and apparent contradictions of adolescent behaviour as stemming from the related processes of *rebellion* and *non-conformity*. The former is particularly apparent if the adolescent faces the need to disengage from over-possessive parents or over-bearing authority, while the latter is a facilitating mechanism which allows adolescents to disengage without undue feelings of guilt or regret. If parents and authority figures can be viewed as old-fashioned and irrelevant, then giving them up becomes more logical and less painful.

Baittle and Offer (1971) point out that non-conformity often takes the form of negation. Whatever those in authority require or demand of the adolescent, he or she wants to do exactly the opposite. Thus the authors argue that in a sense non-conformity is a kind of negative dependency. The adolescent's likes and dislikes, motivations and behaviours, are still dependent upon parents and in part formed by them, but now in a negative sense. Adolescents still lack the confidence to think freely for themselves, but instead of following the lead offered by parents, they now set off determinedly in the opposite direction.

Although based primarily upon clinical insights, and thus not necessarily representative of the whole range of adolescent experience, there is no doubt that the psychoanalytical model does appear to explain some of the excesses and contradictions of adolescent behaviour. The need for independence, and to find and confirm a new adult identity, is clearly a feature of the transition from child to man or woman. However, the way in which this need is satisfied is partly socially-dependent, and in the case of individuals who have been encouraged from an early age to take responsibility for their own behaviour and to exercise independence, there seems no inner psychological imperative condemning the adolescent years to emotional storm and stress.

## The sociological model

Sociological theory recognises the truth of this, and lays particular emphasis upon the social context in which adolescence takes place. The more complex

the social context, and the more conflicting the demands, expectations, opportunities, value-systems and temptations to which adolescents are exposed, the
more likely they are to suffer role conflict and inner doubts and uncertainties.
Marsland (1987) and others place especial emphasis upon the peer group,
which they see as legitimising the adolescent's break with early authority, and
providing him or her with a corporate environment within which to work out
problems of identity and role transition.

In the western world, the breakdown of traditional guidelines is seen by
sociologists as putting particular strains upon the adolescent (Brake 1985). The
decay of the influence of the extended family, of the church, and of the local
community means that the adolescent no longer has a clearly-defined set of
social structures within which to orientate him or herself, and thus is increasingly open to the influence of peers, of the media, of consumerism and of
transient and value-free fashions.

The problem with the sociological theory is that it stems from a broad
perspective of social forces and social behaviours, and thus may tell us little
about the position of individuals. Overall, there is indeed a decay in the modern
world of certain of those social forces which may at one time have served to
provide the adolescent with positive guidance as to behaviour and role. There
is also an increase of violence and of anti-social behaviour, and it would be
strange if this was not reflected in a greater incidence of dissaffection and
lawlessness among the young. But research does not support the idea that in
western cultures most adolescents go through an extreme period of rebellion
against parents and others in authority.

It is true that the incidence of disputes within families tends to peak in early
adolescence (approximately 11 to 15 years), but these disputes typically centre
around minor issues such as household chores, untidiness, homework, noise,
personal appearance, and curfews (Smetana 1988; Steinberg 1987). By late
adolescence, things are calmer. Compromise tends to prevail, largely because
parents see the need to give their growing adolescent children more autonomy,
while the adolescents themselves settle into a more mature relationship with
the adults in their lives. It seems that once autonomy is assured, much of the
need for rebellion disappears (which lends some support to the psychoanalytical
concept of disengagement).

Macoby and Martin (1983) point out that, not surprisingly, parents who
employ domestic democracy, who progressively relax parental discipline, and
who are prepared to negotiate decisions and provide explanations for their own
behaviour, experience fewer problems with their adolescent offspring than do
parents who take a more authoritarian stance, and/or who themselves have a
psychological need to keep their children young and dependent. Thus it may
well be that the sociological perspective is too broad. Adolescent behaviour is
indeed socially dependent to a significant degree, but it is the micro-world of

the family that provides the most important social context, rather than the macro-world of society at large. It seems safe to conclude that wise and enlightened parenting remains, as it has probably always done, of more consequence than any other single social variable.

## The biological model

To psychoanalytical and sociological models of adolescence, we can add the biological model, which takes the view that the undoubtedly extensive and powerful biological changes occuring during the adolescent years lead almost inevitably to a period of conflict and anarchy. Reasoning of this kind was first advanced by Hall back in 1904, when he formulated the idea that ontogeny recapitulates phylogeny – that each individual passes through (recapitulates) the stages in the evolutionary development of the human race itself. Thus in adolescence the individual is at the evolutionary stage of tribal warfare and barbarism that characterised our ancestors, and must, like our ancestors, progress to the stage of civilised and fully socialised behaviour.

Few people take this early view seriously any longer, but biological theorists still adhere to the notion that the physical changes taking place during adolescence (in particular sexual development) produce, in and of themselves, an emotional instability which manifests itself in disturbance and rebellion (Sorenson 1973). Not only do these changes produce instability of mood, they also surprise (and sometimes overwhelm) the adolescent with their intensity, leaving him or her troubled and defensive. Loves and hates become stronger then ever before, and sometimes can only be expressed through anger and violence.

The same new intensity accompanies the advent of sexual maturity. Sexual energy tends to peak in the young male between the ages of 16 and 18, and female sexuality also strengthens powerfully during these years. Sexual desire can therefore become a major preoccupation, often overriding other concerns, and influencing the intensity of personal relationships. In the absence of the moral guidelines that once governed sexual behaviour, many adolescents are unsure of how to behave, or are drawn into sexual activity before they are emotionally mature enough to handle the implications involved. Recent research (Centres for Disease Control 1992) indicates that in the US three quarters of both males and females currently experience pre-marital sexual intercourse, and a sizeable percentage of this activity takes place during the adolescent years.

A further complication arising from biological changes is the rapid alteration in physical appearance that takes place at puberty. The transformation that moves the individual from childhood to a mature adult capable of sexual reproduction takes only some three or four short years (see, for example, Tanner

1970 for full details). It encompasses the adolescent growth spurt (starting around age 12 in girls and two years later in boys), the development of secondary sexual characteristics (breast development in girls, beards in boys, pubic hair in both sexes), and the ripening to full maturity of the primary sex characteristics (the internal and external organs of reproduction).

Particular problems arise when a boy or girl goes through these physical changes much earlier or later than their peers. Petersen (1988) produces results which show that such early or late development (and in some cases even the changes associated with puberty themselves) does have a significant influence upon adolescent self-image, moods, and relationship with parents, peers, and members of the opposite sex. In the case of early maturation (one year ahead of the norm), negative effects appear to be more marked in girls than in boys. Early maturing boys tend to be more satisfied with their appearance than are early maturing girls. The height and strength advantage of early maturing boys over their peers (together perhaps with their earlier initiation into the mystique of manhood) tends to give them prestige and feelings of power. Early maturing girls, by contrast, tend to be embarrassed by their more womanly shape, particularly if breast and hip development is especially marked.

There are of course many individual exceptions to findings of this kind, but they do point to the general psychological impact that the sudden physical changes consequent upon puberty have upon the young. Other studies, such as those by Brooks-Gunn and Ruble (1983), and by Simmons and Blyth (1988) appear to show that early maturing boys have more positive moods than do their pre-pubertal peers, whereas for girls early maturity seems more often to bring depression, lowered self-esteem, and impaired peer and family relationships.

Obviously, many of these feelings about body image are socially conditioned. In a society that favours height and strength in boys, and slimness and agility in girls, it is understandable that boys adapt more readily to the physical changes consequent upon early puberty than do girls. If society changed its image of what was physically desirable, the picture could well change in response. But the other aspect of the biological model, that is, that hormonal and other changes *per se* lie behind many of the emotional and other upsets in adolescents, is more difficult to assess. In an early study, Mead (1928) drew attention to the virtual absence of adolescent problems in the more natural and uncomplicated environment of Samoa. Her research suggested that from the age of five or six onwards, the child increasingly participated in adult tasks, and this participation developed in an orderly and harmonious fashion right up until the child attained full adult rights. Thus, far from being a period of storm and stress, adolescence was a welcome period for all concerned, since it marked the final stage of the process to adult life.

There have been various defences and criticisms of Mead's work (see, for instance, Freeman 1984) over the years, and it does seem that she took a rather too rosy outsider's view of Samoan society. In particular, she appears to have gained much of her information from talking to Samoan women and girls, rather than from talking to both sexes or (better still) observing behaviour. However, her work still carries interest, and does tend to count against the idea that the biological changes resulting from puberty inevitably make adolescence a difficult period for adolescents themselves, and for the elders with whom they relate.

Further support for this comes from Bandura (1972), one of the fathers of modern social psychology, who observed non-problem adolescents (i.e. adolescents who had not been referred for psychological counselling) within their families, and found that the majority of them showed little sign of marked opposition to their parents' values, and little evidence of rebellion or hostility. In the main, adolescence seemed for them to be a time for developing greater trust in, and a more stable relationship with, their parents. On the strength of his findings, Bandura argued that adolescence does not mark an abrupt transition from childhood to adulthood. Throughout childhood, and particularly during the immediate pre-adolescent years, most individuals are increasing their autonomy, so that by puberty it is an already well-established fact. Much of the adjustment in behaviour that remains to be accomplished is on the part of the parents rather than of the children, so that in effect one might talk about parent rather than adolescent problems during the years concerned.

Bandura also challenged another part of the received sociological wisdom of adolescence, namely that the peer group is of such importance that the adolescent conforms indiscrimately to its norms. His findings showed that most adolescents appear to be very choosy about their peer group and about their role models. There was little evidence that adolescents slavishly transferred their psychological dependence from parents to peers. Such a view seemed to do scant justice to the adolescent's growing sense of personal responsibility.

More recently Coleman and Hendry (1990) have cast further doubts upon both the biological and the sociological models, pointing out that the misleading emphasis upon adolescent rebellion and rejection of parental authority is largely a consequence of media misrepresentation on the one hand, and of clinical studies on the other. The media has discovered that adolescent problems make good box-office, while clinical studies have based their findings upon an unrepresentative sample of individuals who come under scrutiny only because of prior psychological problems.

## The cognitive model

Closely linked in some ways to the biological theory is the notion that adolescence sees a final stage in the development of the individual's powers of cognition. This developmental model is associated primarily with the work of Piaget (e.g. 1952), whose research suggested that from infancy onwards our powers of thinking go through a number of progressively more sophisticated and enabling stages, culminating in the stage of *formal operations*, which opens the way to complex abstract thought. Piaget suggested that not all individuals attain formal operations, but that the usual age at which this attainment takes place is early adolescence.

There is no need to go into the Piagetian model in any detail, partly because it is so well described in so many places elsewhere (for example, Flavell 1985). But in brief, it suggests that the abstract thinking that is a major feature of formal operations allows the individual for the first time to explore fully such concepts as justice, values, rights, beliefs, and the whole range of morality and moral behaviour (see also Kohlberg 1969). This can lead to an intense period of questioning and idealism, during which the adolescent supposes he or she has the answer to most of the major problems facing the human race, and may behave impatiently and hyper-critically towards parents, teachers, and other adults.

What often happens at this time is that the adolescent becomes locked into theories. Without the experience of the world and the practical understanding that comes with experience, the adolescent may be unaware of the obstacles that stand in the way of his or her ideals, and may also be unaware that parents and teachers have often gone through exactly the same patterns of thinking that to him or her now appear so original and earth-shattering. Adolescents respond best at this time to wise adults who are able to recognise the importance of idealism, however impractical, at this stage of life, and who are ready to take part in informed and sensible debate. Opposition to adolescent idealism, or attempts to ridicule it, may prompt not only a rebellious response, but may do damage to the adolescent's self-image. In spite of apparent evidence to the contrary, this self-image is often still fragile, and vulnerable to negative adult judgements.

In spite of the doubts that have arisen over the years about the nature and invariability of Piaget's stages of cognitive development, there seems little doubt that adolescents are generally able to think much more effectively at abstract levels than they were hitherto. Thus for the first time they can fully address important issues affecting human equity, well-being and harmony, and can identify weaknesses and errors in the way in which adults run the world. No attempt to understand adolescence would be complete without a realisation of this fact, and no relationship with adolescents is likely to be fully effective that does not take it properly into account.

## The identity model

A strand of thinking that runs through each of the above models is the perceived need during adolescence to change from a child-based to an adult-based identity, whether this is done abruptly or gradually. Erikson (1968) in fact considered that the search for identity marked the final developmental task faced by the individual in the pre-adult years. Failure to accomplish this task successfully led in his view to a sense of role confusion, which left the individual with a diffused identity, likely to be overwhelmed by choices and expectations, and unable to develop a consistent inner self.

Clearly we need at each stage of life to have a coherent sense of who we are, of what we want from life, of what we feel in given situations, of what we can give to others, of what choices we should make. With increased responsibility, this need for an integrated sense of self becomes of ever greater importance, both at a personal and at a social level, and adolescence is one of the episodes when responsibilities rapidly increase (it is not the only period; marriage, parenthood, career progress can all bring comparable or even greater changes in life circumstances).

One undoubted problem often faced by modern adolescents is an absence of appropriate role models to provide a lead in the formulation of a sense of adult identity (Mead 1972). In settled agrarian communities, where skills, values and behaviour changed slowly, parents and other adults provided examples of ways of being which were likely to remain valid for many years to come. In a modern technological society, changes in work, leisure and social demands take place so rapidly that older members of society quickly appear out-of-date in their ideas and levels of expertise. Undoubtedly, this makes the process of identity formation more difficult for the young. Where are they to find their role models, when fashions and marketable skills change so frequently and so dramatically?

Erikson considered that there are four problems facing the adolescent in his or her search for identity, the needs for *intimacy*, for an appropriate *time perspective*, for *industry*, and to avoid the development of a *negative identity*. Intimacy refers to the ability not just to form close relationships with others, but to do so without losing a sense of personal identity. One needs to be able to love others by being oneself, not by moulding oneself eternally to their expectations. Time perspective refers to the ability to look and plan ahead, and to operate within a realistic time scale. If the individual is afraid of change, or too anxious for change, then he or she will either try to cling to the *status quo*, or to attempt an impossible achievement timetable, and end up disappointed and disillusioned with self and others.

Industry means the ability to work productively and with due commitment, and to make appropriate and informed choices between all the various tasks that may be clamouring for attention. All too often the adolescent proves unable to set priorities, or to complete an individual task before turning, out of anxiety or boredom, to another. Finally, the avoidance of a negative identity means much the same as avoidance of the extreme non-conformity to which reference was made under the psychoanalytical model. A negative identity arises not from positive decisions about the person one wishes to be, but out of the desire to be as unlike others as possible. Trapped within a negative identity, the individual forfeits his or her existential freedom, and is as much dependent upon others in a negative sense as in early childhood he or she was dependent upon them in a positive way.

As with the other models, the identity model seems by no means applicable in all cases. Siddique and D'Arcy (1984) found indications of an identity crisis in only one quarter of their large sample of adolescents. And it seems likely that a similar percentage would be found even in adult groups at important transitional stages in life. We are all of us unsure of who we are when the markers by which we orientate ourselves and our lives – whether these markers have to do with relationships, our profession, or even our physical environment – suddenly disappear or are significantly altered in some way.

For example, the lifespan approach of Lerner (1985) suggests that people at all stages of their lives play an active role in creating their environment. Rather than being victims of circumstances, adolescents, as much as individuals within other age groups, thus have the potential to interact with the people and events in their lives in ways that positively shape both the environment and their own personal development. Lerner's model proposes that this inter-action typically goes through three episodes. In the first of these, the adolescent evokes through his or her behaviour reactions from others (supportive, angry, directive etc. depending upon personal and social variables); he or she then processes the information provided by these reactions and tries to make sense of it in terms of current levels of understanding (episode two); finally, the adolescent acts as a positive agent by choosing, shaping and selecting future interactions (episode three). The more autonomous the adolescent, the more likely he or she is to progress through all three episodes, and to do so in an appropriate and enriching way.

## The focal model

Each of the above models therefore has something to offer in our understanding of adolescence, but none of them seems adequate in itself. As with other psychological models, they each suffer from the weakness that they attempt to provide an all-inclusive pattern to which all individuals, regardless of their temperament, their relationships, their circumstances and their prior experience are expected to conform. One of the great features of humankind is the diversity that exists between individuals, and this diversity is as apparent in adolescence as it is at all other times of life. Human beings defy precise categorisation, and any attempt to impose it upon them risks reducing them to two-dimensional caricatures of themselves.

One model that attempts to combine many of the features of the various models discussed so far, and which resists setting apart adolescents and their problems from other stages of human life, is the focal theory advanced by Coleman. In the course of his research (Coleman and Hendry 1990), Coleman has explored the manner in which anxieties, interests, self-image, friendships etc. change during the years from 11 through to 17. Results indicate that as individuals pass through adolescence, their attention becomes focused on different aspects of their lives. Once one set of issues is resolved, they recede into the background, and the focus of attention changes to something else. This does not mean that adolescents pass sequentially through the major challenges and problems of their lives, simply that all are not equally important at any one time. Real difficulties occur only when many of the challenges are present in equal strength, and the individual becomes overloaded and unable to deal with each focus separately.

Overload of this kind may stretch the adolescent beyond the limits of his or her coping strategies, and take away the freedom of choice. Ideally, the individual should be able to decide which challenge needs maximum focus at any one time, and attend to that secure in the knowledge that others areas of life are currently stable and relatively stress-free.

The advantage of this model is that it sees all the concerns highlighted by other models of adolescence as providing potential points of focus. Thus disengagement from parents may be a focus at one time; sociological and peer group pressures at another; body image and sexual development at another; relationships with the opposite sex at another; identity, career choice and life goals at another; values and beliefs at another and so on. The weakness of the model is that it can tell us nothing about the individual's ability to cope with each area of focus, or about his or her psychological resilience in dealing with focus overload. Like all models, it is in some sense an abstraction which, for all its neatness, may not be an accurate reflection of how the adolescent actually experiences life.

Do individuals at this stage in fact see themselves as primarily a focus-orientated process? Does such a process accurately represent their self-image, or their growing sense of adult identity? Where the model does score, of course, is that it helps us, when working with or counselling adolescents, to explore with them the nature of their areas of focus and determine whether there is overload or confusion between these areas or whether one area is being concentrated upon to the exclusion of other, potentially more important, ones. Thus at a cognitive level we can help them think more coherently about their lives, and plan present and future behaviour with more care and insight.

## Conclusion

An understanding of the problems of adolescence requires us to have a good working knowledge of each of the above models, and of the way in which each can elucidate some part of the trials and challenges faced by individuals during this period of life. But we need a further level of understanding, namely that adolescents are individuals, and that we must be wary of over-generalising about them. Allied to this, we need to accept that adolescence is not a period of life separate from any other, but part of a continuous process that presents the individual with recurring challenges and opportunities from early childhood through into old age.

As for the future, the only thing that one can say with certainty is that these challenges and opportunities will continue, with a rapidly changing environment exacerbating some and diminishing others. The speed of technological change and the likely continuing decline of traditional values and moral codes are the two factors most likely to exacerbate problems, while the further opening up of educational opportunities is likely to be the prime factor behind the diminution of others. One thing however is clear: adolescence is always likely to remain a major focus of media attention, and an important target for adult concern and disapproval. It was indeed ever thus. Even the ancient Greeks lamented the falling standards of the young. And in the readiness of each generation to disapprove of the behaviour of the next we have a psychological phenomenon which in itself is worthy of serious research attention.

## References

Baittle, B. and Offer, D. (1971) 'On the nature of adolescent rebellion.' In F.C. Feinstein, P. Giovacchini and A. Miller (eds) *Annals of Adolescent Psychiatry.* New York: Basic Books.

Bandura, A. (1972) 'The stormy decade: fact or fiction?' In D. Rogers (ed) *Issues in Adolescent Psychology,* (2nd edn). New York: Appleton-Century-Crofts.

Blos, P. (1967) 'The second individuation process of adolescence.' *Psychoanalytical Study of the Child 22,* 162–186.

Brake, M. 1985) *Comparative Youth Sub-Cultures.* London: Routledge and Kegan Paul.

Brooks-Gunn, J. and Ruble, D.N. (1983) 'The experience of menarche from a developmental perspective.' In J. Brooks-Gunn and A.C. Petersen (eds) *Girls at Puberty: Biological and Psychological Perspectives.* New York: Plenum.

Centers for Disease Control (1992) 'Sexual behaviour among high school students, United States 1990.' *Morbidity and Mortality Weekly Report 40,* 885–888.

Coleman, J.C. (1994) 'Adolescence.' In A.M. Colman (ed) *Companion Encyclopedia of Psychology 2.* London: Routledge.

Coleman, J.C. and Hendry, L. (1990) *The Nature of Adolescence,* (2nd edition). London: Routledge.

Erikson, E. (1968) *Identity: Youth and Crisis.* New York: Norton.

Flavell, J.H. (1985) *Cognitive Development*, (2nd edition). Englewood Cliffs NJ: Prentice-Hall.

Freeman, D. (1984) *Margaret Mead and Samoa: the Making and Unmaking of an Anthropological Myth*. Harmondsworth: Penguin.

Hall, G.C. (1904) *Adolescence*. New York: Appleton.

Kohlberg, L. (1969) *Stages in Development of Moral Thought and Action*. New York: Holt, Rinehart and Winston.

Lerner, R.M. (1985) 'Adolescent maturational changes and psychosocial development: a dynamic interactional perspective.' *Journal of Youth and Adolescence 3*, 7–16.

Lerner, R.M. (1987) In V.B. Van Hasselt and M. Herson (eds) *Handbook of Adolescent Psychology*. Oxford: Pergamon.

Maccoby, E.E. and Martin, J.A. (1983) 'Socialization in the context of the family: parent–child interaction.' In P.H. Mussen (ed) *Handbook of Child Psychology 4*. New York: Wiley.

Marsland, D. (1987) *Education and Youth*. London: Falmer.

Mead, M. (1928) *Coming of Age in Samoa*. (1970 edition) Harmondsworth: Penguin.

Mead, M. (1972) *Culture and Commitment*. St. Albans: Panther.

Peterson, A.C. (1988) 'Adolescent development.' In M.R. Rosenzweig and L.W. Porter (eds) *Annual Review of Psychology 39*. Palo Alto: Annual Reviews.

Piaget, J. (1952) *The Origins of Intelligence in Children. New York: International Universities Press.*

Siddique, C.M. and D'Arcy, C. (1984) 'Adolescence, stress and psychological wellbeing.' *Journal of Youth and Adolescence 13*, 459–474.

Simmons, R.G. and Blyth D.A. (1988) *Moving into Adolescence: The Impact of Pubertal Change and School Context*. New York: Aldine.

Smetana, J.G. (1988) 'Concepts of self and social convention: adolescents' and parents' reasoning about hypothetical and actual family conflicts.' In M.R. Gunnar and W.A. Collins (eds) *The Minnesota Symposium 21*. Hillsdale NJ: Erlbaum.

Sorenson, R.C. (1973) *Adolescent Sexuality in Contemporary America*. New York: World.

Steinberg, L. (1987) 'Impact of puberty on family relations. Effects of pubertal status and pubertal timing.' *Developmental Psychology 23*, 451–460.

Tanner, J.M. (1970) 'Physical growth.' In P.H. Mussen (ed) *Carmichael Manual of Child Psychology Vol I*, (3rd edition). New York: Wiley.

# CHAPTER 8

# Depression in Childhood and Adolescence

*Margaret Wright*

## Introduction

It was originally thought that the clinical state of depression did not occur in childhood or adolescence. This is not true. Children and adolescents are not immune to this illness. Indeed the manual of Mental Disorders (DSM III R) now recognises this fact; it states clearly that the features of mood disorder are the same in children as in adults and the special categories are not given seperately in the section belonging to children and adolescence in the manual (in adults the special categories include a single episode of major depression, recurrent major depressions and depressive neurosis). This represents an enormous leap forward from the beginning of recognition of this illness in the 1970s.

It was originally Dr Eva Frommer working in St Thomas's Hospital, Westminster, who recognised the illness in her patients and started writing articles about it. She was adamant that some persistent disorders of a developmental, emotional, or behavioural nature had an underlying biological cause and was the first doctor to acknowledge publicly that antidepressants had an important role in the treatment of this disorder and that results helped to prove this observation. Previously it had been regarded as sufficient to label problems in adolescents as developmental delays, aggressive outbursts, school refusal, sphincter disorders, phobias and other disorders. Psychological and sociological explanations were considered sufficient to explain the origin of such problems. The presence of a biochemical change in neuro-endocrine underlying and causing these outward manifestations was postulated instead. This immediately allied it to the already acknowledged depressions widely recognised in adults. Of course the representations and manifestations are markedly different in adolescents.

also the positive effect of diminishing the difficulties and failures that depression can produce in the behaviour for their teachers and their work output. Such acquired criticism of their work output diminishes their self-esteem and adds to their feeling of worthlessness. It is important to explain to teachers that their pupil would do better if they were able. Their temporary difficulty to perform well is outside their present control, but will return. Similarly, competitive or an extra demanding situation can cause too much distress so should be avoided if possible.

These children desperately need a special sort of sympathetic attention. This includes opportunities for more rest, extra loving attention to simple needs and the removal of any hostility that their change of behaviour has caused in others. It must be pointed out that a depressed child or adolescent behaves in a way that does not elicit the normal responses from anyone; instead they are more likely to receive reactions of exasperation, impatience or even anger from any carer. This is when a reminder should be given that the child is unable to function normally at present and cannot manage good behaviour and be their normal loveable self.

It is important to tempt them with nutritious food of their own liking. Any creative tasks should only be undertaken if the child wants them or is familiar with the techniques already. Sometimes their whole behaviour can be regressed temporarily and they adopt childish attributes. They may select childish toys and books destined for the younger children because they are familiar. To expect the children to strive and achieve new targets only produces new opportunities for failure and hopelessness.

Family therapy has a role here to clarify and possibly reorganise power structures to allow healthy interactions between parents and siblings. Parents will become ready to clarify any unhelpful contribution from within their nuclear family to help the victim who is beginning to show improvement in their illness. The aim is always to prevent anyone from being scapegoated. These unshared, previously hidden difficulties can be allowed to surface and receive clarification. Remedies are sought which are comfortable and acceptable for everyone.

Antidepressants may be of use but it is important to explain that an antidepressant will not produce an improvement for at least a week. Medication is not normally continued for longer than six weeks and the dosage can be tailed off slowly. The medication is not addictive and it is rarely necessary to order second courses. My choice is a sedative tricyclic drug which is given as a solitary dose at night time according to the body weight of the child or adolescent.

Above all, the aim of any help must be for the patient to begin to regain their own self-esteem and feel better. This comes when their energy level improves and the renewed experience of their inner well-being exerts itself.

This is reinforced by remarks from carers and doctors who say that 'he or she is more like themselves now'. The greatest joy is when they can smile and their sense of humour returns. Present activities give them pleasure and they look forward to a bright future too.

## Prognosis

Childhood depressions need not recur. It is to be hoped that the children or adolescents have learnt from their experience new strategies to deal with any stressful events in their lives. They can learn not to personalise blame when things happen which are not of their making. They learn to express their feelings verbally about events and share reactions as they happen with a confiding adult. No longer should they internalise events making them destructive to their well-being. Instead they are able to find ways of balancing actions with positive reactions. Good memories of experiences from the past can be allowed to surface so that they can face the future differently and optimistically.

An unrecognised and therefore untreated depression can have the aspects of helplessness and the resulting poor self-image incorporated into the developing personality. The reversal of this demands massive changes in relationships and environment which affect everyone involved.

## Conclusion

The signalling of a depression asks for a change of attitude from their onlookers and possibly a call for clemency. So a depressive illness can offer a shell or protection from adversity, or an escape from a lifestyle that produces suffering that is intolerable. In ethological terms we can observe an element of passivity in all the symptoms and signs which is like that of animals, whose crawling or cowering away may be a sign of submission to ward off aggressive attacks.

There are various factors during the early development of a child that can provide protection against these depressive episodes. The most important must be the early nurturing experiences and attachment provided by their caring adult. This is when any discomfort or pressing needs are responded to by the loving relationship from mother or her substitute.

To be of maximum value this response must be reliable, consistent and regular. In this way an infant learns that he can exchange a bad experience for a good warm human response. This piece of learning must represent the beginning of an understanding about metaphors. It fits the definition of a metaphor which is: a descriptive term or phrase for an object or action to which it is imaginatively but not literally applicable. It leaves the child with a healing experience given from love by another person. This feeds and increases his or her internal well-being and safety. This healthy effect outlasts any disaster; it allows the new growth of the personality following a painful experience.

Nearly 500 years ago William Shakespeare wrote his introductory speech for Antonio in his play *The Merchant of Venice:*

> In sooth, I know not why I am so sad;
> It wearies me; you say it wearies you;
> But, how I caught it, found it, or came by it,
> What stuff, 'tis made of, where of it is born,
> I am to learn;
> And such a want-wit sadness makes of me
> That I have much ado to know myself.

What is depression? How can we explain its occurrence and persistence in human misery? Many questions remain but I have given you my own thoughts and knowledge from a professional lifetime working with troubled children and adolescents.

# CHAPTER 9

# Troubles of Learning

*Howard Roberts*

## Introduction

Academic failure can be devastating for children. Success is often equated with self worth and there is a risk that those who fail will feel themselves to be of little value. However, it is important that this overvaluation of success does not lead us to undervalue its importance. Academic success at school is important and quite rightly political parties have put the issue to the top of their agenda. Children are tested regularly during their time at school. Schools are ranked by exam results in league tables and there is a widespread view that our educational system is not achieving what it should or could. However, there is little agreement as to what, if anything, has gone wrong. Culprits vary; some people blame parents, others teachers, some society, others schools and some individual children. Clearly, there is no simple explanation for such a complex problem and numerous factors contribute to a child's success or otherwise at school. Rather than try to cover the whole area, in this chapter I intend to focus on one issue which is sometimes overlooked. Academic failure often occurs in association with child mental health problems (Chazan and Laing 1994). Croll and Moses (1985) reported that more than two thirds of children with emotional and behavioural problems had difficulties with their learning. As 7.7 per cent of the children in their survey were identified as having problems of this kind the numbers of children involved was large. It is important that we understand the relationship between these two otherwise there is a danger that a vicious circle will be created whereby one exacerbates the other and this is the issue I will be considering in this chapter.

Before I do this I will discuss some general matters related to psychiatric problems in children. First we need to consider the issue of classification. Not all are agreed about the usefulness of making psychiatric diagnoses. On the one hand there has been much interest recently in attempting to refine the clinical psychiatric syndromes so that issues such as the aetiology, treatment and prognosis of child mental health problems can be investigated and some go so far as to say that in the past our understanding has been hindered by the fact that psychiatric diagnoses have sometimes not been made. However, others do not think that child mental health problems should be classified. In their view each child needs to be considered as an individual in his own right and they think that grouping children together in terms of their symptoms distracts attention from the individual child's emotional needs and problems.

## Why classify?

The merits and demerits of classification have recently been clearly and concisely discussed by Cantwell and Rutter (1994). According to this view we classify everything and classification is merely a way of ordering information. The important issue is not whether we classify but how we classify and this depends on what we are trying to achieve with our classification. Thus, mental health problems in children can be classified in many different but equally valid ways for example in terms of the child's social environment, family pathology or by psychiatric diagnosis. Classification is not therefore an uncovering of reality, but a structuring of it for certain purposes.

## What are the advantages of classification by psychiatric diagnosis?

Some agree that classification is needed but argue that classifying by psychiatric diagnosis incorrectly locates the problem within the child whereas in reality the child is either a victim of adverse social circumstances or a participant in a pathological system or that at the very least the child's problems should be seen as the result of a mismatch between the child and his environment or as an understandable reaction to his environment (e.g. Furlong 1993; Cooper, Smith and Upton 1994). Cooper et al. (1994) point out that if the problems are thought to reside within the child, the implication is that it is the child who must be treated and cured and they think that in the case of behavioural problems 'the tendency to focus attention solely on the individual pupil' (p.20)… 'removes the need to question the value of the school structures and regimes' (p.21). However, psychiatric diagnoses are descriptions of symptoms. They do not in themselves tell us anything about how the symptoms are caused and classification by psychiatric diagnosis does not preclude the use of other classifications. All agree that psychiatric problems are due to an interaction between the child and his environment and that an understanding of the child's social circumstances are crucial to understanding their psychiatric problems. Each child has his own unique biology and psychology and different children react differently to the same environmental stress. Psychiatric diagnosis helps us to understand the significance of a particular environment for a particular child. Nowadays, the general view amongst child psychiatrists is that a combination of both symptoms and impairment gives the most meaningful diagnosis (Cantwell and Rutter 1994).

In addition, as the psychiatric diagnosis is based on descriptions of symptoms the disorders can be operationally defined and, as it avoids consideration of theoretical issues about how symptoms are formed, it can be used by individuals with different views to investigate aetiologies without any presuppositions being made. Comparisons between workers can be made and communication is enhanced. Clearly, the descriptions used should have clinical relevance and should for example have implications for treatment or prognosis.

## How are child mental health problems classified?

In both of the main classifications in use, the International Classification of Diseases (ICD) and the Diagnostic and Statistical Manual of Mental Disorders (DSM) the psychiatric diagnosis is made on several axes. This multiaxial approach is an attempt to give clinical meaning to the diagnosis by adding relevant contextual factors. The latest edition of the DSM (DSM4) includes five axes (see Table 9.1).

### Table 9.1 Axes included in DSM4

| | |
|---|---|
| Axis 1 | Clinical diagnosis |
| Axis 2 | Mental retardation/personality disorder |
| Axis 3 | General medical conditions |
| Axis 4 | Psychosocial/environmental problems |
| Axis 5 | Global assessment/functioning |

The DSM 4 is described in detail elsewhere (DSM 41994). Briefly, the clinical diagnosis such as Major Depressive Disorder, Attention Deficit Disorder etc. is included in Axis 1. The purpose of the other axes is to make sure that issues which are relevant to the Axis 1 diagnosis are not overlooked. Thus, the child's IQ and a description of his personality and the defence mechanisms used are included on Axis 2; current general medical conditions are included on Axis 3; Axis 4 includes relevant environmental factors; and Axis 5 is for giving a summary assessment of the overall level of the individual's functioning. This is useful in gauging the significance of the Axis 1 diagnosis and in planning treatment and predicting prognosis. There are guidelines indicating how impairment of functioning should be assessed.

In the remainder of this chapter I will describe four common and important psychiatric problems and consider the links between these and academic difficulties at school.

## 1. Conduct disorder/oppositional disorder

The child with Conduct Disorder presents with antisocial behaviour. There is disagreement about how this condition should be conceptualised but all are agreed that it is a serious problem with a poor long-term prognosis. Research has shown that about half of the children with Conduct Disorder become adults with antisocial problems and many of the remainder develop other psychiatric difficulties in adult life.

Conduct Disorder needs to be considered from several different vantage points and family, school, community and characteristics of the individual all contribute to the problem. However, there have been suggestions that the school environment may be of particular importance. For example, Offord, Boyle and Racine (1991) reported that many children with Conduct Disorder were identified only by teachers and they thought that this might be because the school environment is particularly relevant to the problem.

Children with Conduct Disorder present with behavioural problems, aggression and truancy and it is therefore unlikely that they will be overlooked by the teacher. As they often have a low verbal IQ and academic problems such as reading retardation and there is a tendency to under-perform at school relative to their peers, these children are likely to find the school environment particularly stressful and it may be for this reason that they are more likely to show symptoms at school. However, in some cases children with Conduct Disorder have symptoms at home and are well-behaved at school. These children sometimes come from socially deprived backgrounds and from families where there is poor parenting, sometimes with physical abuse. The parents often fail to set appropriate standards and monitor the child's behaviour so that fitting into the regime at school and co-operating with their peers might be difficult for them. In a discussion of the causes of academic failure in these children Earls (1994) concluded that both the Conduct Disorder and the low verbal IQ are probably caused by social factors, possibly an impoverished home environment.

These children may show cognitive problems in social relationships and are more likely to misinterpret the intentions of others as hostile, are less good at solving social problems and have fewer social skills. They are therefore more likely to try to resolve difficulties with others by using violence. From a clinical point of view these children often give the impression of having difficulties in finding a way of gaining recognition from others, other than by being aggressive and domineering, and have few ways of dealing with frustration other than by violent antisocial behaviour.

The most effective approach to prevention and treatment seems to be one that combines a programme which enables the child to acquire skills, which need not necessarily be academic, with exposure to non-deviant peers, who can act as role models and with opportunities for learning socially acceptable behaviour by positive reinforcement from the parents. It is also useful to help the child become more sensitive in interpersonal situations and to help them find ways of solving problems involving social conflict. Clearly, the school has a major role to play in this. School is likely to be a very challenging environment for these children because of their academic difficulties and because of the many opportunities for social conflict which will need resolution. There may be a cultural gap between the standards of behaviour and discipline expected at school and the expectations at home.

## 2. Attention deficit hyperactivity disorder (ADHD)

ADHD is a disorder characterised by inattention, difficulty in concentrating, distractibility, impulsiveness, restlessness and over-activity. The problem is probably under-diagnosed in this country and is more common in boys than girls. The teacher often becomes aware of the problem in the early school years but the parents may have had concerns before the child started at school. At school there is often difficulty in keeping the child on task. The child finds it difficult to concentrate and falls behind with his work and a cycle of negative attention-seeking behaviour may be established. The child often has problems in his social relationships with his peers and he may be aggressive, domineering, unpopular and socially isolated.

Often there is an associated developmental delay with delayed language development and poor motor co-ordination. Children with ADHD are at increased risk for Conduct Disorder, in which case antisocial behaviour is also present. The presence of a Conduct Disorder worsens the prognosis and, in adolescence, aggression, antisocial behaviour and delinquency may cause serious problems for the child, the teacher and the parents.

At home the parents may complain that the child is always on the go and has difficulty in settling to things. Similar behaviour may be noticed at school although the problem may be situational with the child showing problems in one environment and behaving normally in others.

The learning problems associated with hyperactivity have been discussed in detail by Taylor (1994). He concludes that there is a specific cognitive deficit associated with hyperactivity which is at high executive levels of functioning. This results in children making rapid inaccurate responses in conditions of uncertainty. The problem is not due to their being distracted by extraneous stimuli and it seems as if they can control their responses but do not do so because they have an intense dislike of delay. Following on from this he concludes that the key to effective teaching is not excluding irrelevant stimuli, although no doubt as with any child this is helpful, but that the primary aim should be to keep the child applied to the task.

Some long-term outcome studies have found that the prognosis in a can be surprisingly favourable but the outcome is worse if there is as aggressive behaviour.

Treatment consists of medication, combined with behaviour therapy and educational therapy. Stimulant medication, Methylphenidate, improves the symptoms in the majority of children. The medication can have a dramatic effect on the child and the school may know when the child has not taken his medication by the change in his behaviour. However, about 25 per cent either do not respond to the medication or are made worse. Other medications can be prescribed which may be helpful and behaviour therapy aimed at helping the child attend to their work and helping them control their hyperactive behaviour can be combined with the medication. Educational therapy with a behavioural approach can help the child attend to the tasks in hand and can be used to modify unacceptable behaviour.

## 3. Depression

Clinically significant depression needs to be distinguished from sadness and unhappiness which is a normal emotional response to certain types of events in our lives. In depressive disorders other symptoms are associated with the depressed mood and the individual may report a loss of enjoyment of activities which were previously pleasurable (anhedonia) or may have negative ideas about himself and his world. Some have suicidal ideas.

Depressive disorders are less common in children than adults. They are very uncommon in pre-school children but the frequency increases at school age to about 2.5 per cent. There is a further increase in prevalence in adolescence to around 4.5 per cent and as the adolescent gets older the prevalence increases further to the rate in adults (Kashani and Schmid 1992). Many cases of depression in children and adolescents are undiagnosed and untreated as both parents and teachers are often unaware of the fact that the child is depressed. This is probably at least partly due to the fact that the child has not told the adults about their symptoms (Barrett *et al.* 1991). There are a number of reasons why they may not have reported their symptoms and it does highlight the need to interview the child on his own. The significance of childhood depression varies but the diagnosis is important as it can be associated with considerable morbidity; suicide rates have increased greatly in young people in recent years and depression is a risk factor for suicide (Merikangas and Angst 1995).

The long term prognosis of childhood depression has not been fully worked out but in clinical samples childhood depression does appear to be a chronic condition with a high rate of relapse (Kovacs *et al.* 1984) and follow-up studies indicate that children who attended a clinic with depression in childhood are at greater risk of further episodes in adult life (Harrington *et al.* 1990).

There has been little systematic research into the effects of depression on the performance of children at school. Given that the symptoms include difficulty in concentrating, (Forness 1988; Stark 1990) hopelessness and negative self-evaluations (Stark 1990) one might expect that depressed children would have difficulty in managing their school work. In addition, it is well known that depressed adults have cognitive problems with disturbances of memory, attention and reasoning (Robert and Beau 1995). However, the research on the academic performance of depressed children is not altogether consistent. Depression does appear to be associated with a deterioration in academic performance (Stark 1990) but the mechanisms are not clear. There are a number of possibilities. Depression is associated with school refusal and this will clearly have an impact on school achievement but only a minority of depressed children are school non-attenders. Depressed children do not appear to perform differently from other children on IQ tests and attempts to identify specific difficulties in academic tasks such as reading or maths have not yielded consistent results (Stark 1990; Forness 1988). It has been suggested that depression does not result in a specific profile of academic difficulties, but rather that the poor school performance associated with depression is a result of the depressives' general lack of interest and negative self-evaluation (Stark 1990). Clinically, some depressed children are quiet and withdrawn and do not engage fully in classroom activities and may therefore get overlooked.

Several treatments are used but they have not been fully evaluated. It is clearly important to offer help with any major stress. Psychological treatments include cognitive behaviour therapy which aims to correct current maladaptive thoughts. Social skills training and interpersonal therapy, both of which aim to help with current problems in interpersonal relations, are also used. Although there is good evidence that medication is a valuable treatment for depressed adults, it has not so far been shown to be useful for children although several medications have been introduced in recent years which have not been evaluated.

### 4. Anxiety Disorder

Anxiety is an inevitable part of normal development and only becomes pathological if it is severe or persistent or occurs at an inappropriate age. Infants normally show anxiety during the latter part of the first year, with a fear of strangers and anxiety if they are separated from their caregivers. At age two they often fear strange objects and people, at age three animals and at age four to five the dark. Concerns about performance at school occur later in childhood and social anxieties in adolescence.

Anxiety Disorders are very common in children and most do not have serious implications either with regard to current impairment or long-term prognosis.

Having said this however, it is important not to minimise their significance as anxiety disorders can be very disabling and follow-up studies indicate a continuity with neurotic disorders in later childhood (Richman, Stevenson and Graham 1982) and that around half of adults with anxiety disorders had an onset in childhood.

Separation Anxiety declines with age and only becomes pathological if it is severe and persistent. The child may present with distress on separation from the mother, worries about family members, clinging, school refusal, nightmares and somatic complaints. It may represent a persistence of normal separation or be precipitated by an acute stress or separation at a later age. The symptoms tend to improve with age but may worsen in adolescence when the child takes on additional responsibilities. Many adults with agoraphobia have a history of Separation Anxiety Disorder.

Children with Avoidant Disorder get anxious in the presence of strangers but seek the presence of familiar people. This resembles the stranger anxiety of the seven month old. The child is shy, withdrawn, quiet, may refuse to attend school and so become isolated. Spontaneous improvement is less likely than with Separation Anxiety and it may lead to Social Phobia.

Phobic Anxieties are irrational fears of open or closed spaces, animals, heights, the dark, thunder, school etc. In one study 2.4 per cent of eleven year olds had simple phobias. They may have no other symptoms or may have a diffuse generalised anxiety, an associated depression or school refusal. The phobia may continue into adult life.

Sometimes anxiety is not focused on any particular object or situation. In this case it is called Over-Anxious Disorder and may present with symptoms such as excessive and unrealistic fears, nightmares, loss of self confidence, approval seeking and apprehensiveness, multiple somatic complaints and school refusal. Sometimes the parents are excessively anxious.

Although some children with anxiety disorders are readily identified, research suggests that neither teachers nor parents are good at recognising the anxious child and as a result most go undiagnosed.

Many children with anxiety disorders function within the normal range academically (Stark 1990). However, others attend school erratically and their academic achievements are impaired. The relationship between anxiety disorders and academic performance in children is in need of further research. In a review of the literature Quay and La Greca (1986) reported that highly anxious students performed less well on a number of achievement tasks. Children with test anxiety showed more negative self-evaluations and tended to compare themselves unfavourably with others. They found it more difficult to concentrate and were more distractable. Quay and La Greca thought that these children's expectations of failure were likely to undermine their efforts. It is not clear to what extent these findings also apply to clinical anxiety.

The usefulness of the various treatment options has not been evaluated. Involvement of the family is useful as the child often manipulates the parents into helping them avoid situations that provoke anxiety and this makes the anxiety worse. Behaviour therapy techniques such as relaxation, exposure and reinforcement are also useful. If these fail, medication can be used although its place in the treatment of anxiety disorders of childhood is not established.

In this chapter I have described four psychiatric problems and the effect that they may have on a child's academic performance at school. In doing this I am not suggesting that other issues are not important and neither am I suggesting that a child's mental health problems should be considered in isolation from important environmental factors which impinge on the child, such as the organisation of the school, the educational system or the child's family. The child's mental health is one factor amongst many which need to be considered when we are trying to find out why a child has failed at school.

## References

Barrett, M.L., et al. (1991) 'Diagnosing childhood depression. Who should be interviewed – parent or child?' Depression in Childhood, British Journal of Psychiatry 159, Suppl 11, 22–27.

Cantwell, D.P. and Rutter, M. (1994) 'Classification: conceptual issues and substantive findings.' In M. Rutter, E. Taylor and L. Hersov (eds) Child and Adolescent Psychiatry: Modern Approaches. Oxford: Blackwell.

Chazan, M. and Laing, A.F. (1994) Emotional and Behavioural Difficulties in Middle Childhood. London: Falmer Press.

Cooper, P., Smith, C.T. and Upton, G. (1994) Emotional and Behavioural Difficulties: Theory to Practice. London: Routledge.

Croll, P. and Moses, D. (1985) One in Five: The Assessment and Incidence of Special Educational Needs. London: Routledge and Kegan Paul.

Earls, F. (1994) 'Oppositional defiant and conduct disorders.' In M. Rutter, E. Taylor and L. Hersov (eds) Child and Adolescent Psychiatry: Modern Approaches. Oxford: Blackwell.

Forness, S.R. (1988) 'School characteristics of children and adolescents with depression.' In R.B. Rutherford, C.M. Nelson and S.R. Forness (eds) Bases of Severe Behavioural Disorders in Children and Youth. Boston, Mass: Little, Brown.

Furlong, V.J. (1993) 'Sociological perspectives in disaffection from school.' In V. Varma (ed) Management of Behaviour in Schools. London: Longman.

Harrington, R.D., et al. (1990) 'Adult outcomes of childhood and adolescent depression. 1. psychiatric states.' Archives of General Psychiatry 47, 465–473.

Kashani, J.H. and Schmid, L.S. (1992) 'Epidemiology and aetiology of depressive disorders.' In M. Shafi and S.L. Shafi (eds) Clinical Guide to Depression in Children and Adolescents. Washington, DC: American Psychiatric Press.

Kovacs, M., et al. (1984) 'Depressive disorders in childhood. 11. a longitudinal study of risk for subsequent major depression.' Archives of General Psychiatry 41, 643–649.

Merikangas, K.R. and Angst, J. (1995) 'The challenge of depressive disorders in adolescents.' In M. Rutter (ed) *Psychosocial Disturbances in Young People: Challenges for Prevention.* Cambridge: Cambridge University Press.

Offord, D.R., *et al.* (1991) 'The epidemiology of antisocial behaviour in childhood and adolescence.' In D.J. Pepler and K.H. Rubin (eds) *The Development and Treatment of Childhood Aggression.* Hillsdale, NJ: Lawrence Erlbaum.

Quay, H. and La Greca, A.M. (1986) 'Disorders of anxiety, withdrawal and dysphoria.' In H. Quay and J.S. Werry (eds) *Psychopathological Disorders of Childhood.* New York: John Wiley.

Richman, N., Stevenson, J. and Graham, P.J. (1982) *Preschool to School: A Behavioural Study.* London: Academic Press.

Robert, P.H. and Beau, C.H. (1995) 'Cognitive functioning and therapy for treating depression.' *Focus on Depression 3,* 6–9.

Stark, K.D. (1990) *Childhood Depression. School Based Intervention.* New York: Guilford.

Taylor, E. (1994) 'Syndromes of attention deficit and overactivity.' In M. Rutter, E. Taylor and L. Hersov (eds) *Child and Adolescent Psychiatry: Modern Approaches.* Oxford: Blackwell.

# CHAPTER 10

# Troubles of Discipline

*Robert Povey*

Don't do that
Why not?
'Cos I say so!

Children and adolescents frequently get into trouble with adults whether at school or at home because of so-called 'discipline' problems. This usually means that they have infringed in some way the rules of behaviour which are seen (sometimes only by the adults involved) as applicable to the context in which the behaviour has taken place. 'Disciplined behaviour' thus involves children following some sort of rules, whether these are self-imposed, mutually agreed or set without consultation by an authority figure (*see* Smith 1985). Where the rules are imposed 'from above' without discussion or agreement ('cos I say so') the discipline involves a degree of coercion, often with an implied threat of punishment – 'and if you don't you'll be for it'. This imposed, coercive and punitive type of discipline is sometimes superficially effective in keeping order on a temporary basis. However, it is generally not very effective in producing children and adolescents who possess good self-discipline and a genuine consideration for others. The latter qualities are much more likely to be encouraged by disciplinary approaches in which the emphasis is on the *reinforcement of desired behaviour* (rather than on adult-imposed, punitive penalties) and in which *agreed* rules of behaviour are consistently applied within the context of a warm and accepting family or school environment. Indeed research studies have convincingly demonstrated the effectiveness of strategies which involve children collaborating in the establishment of agreed school rules, even in inner-city schools with a high proportion of severely disadvantaged and behaviourally challenging pupils (see Docking 1993).

In the first part of the chapter I shall examine general approaches to discipline at home and at school and this will be followed by consideration of the use of behaviour-modification techniques as an aid to maintaining classroom discipline. The chapter ends with a discussion of bullying in the classroom and an examination of the problems associated with the exclusion of disruptive pupils from school. Illustrative case studies are included in each section.

### Discipline at home

The same broad principles apply to questions of 'discipline' whether these involve children at home or at school. There are some differences, of course, in the way in which discipline matters are handled because of the different settings involved – parents rather than teachers, one or two offspring as opposed to large classes of unrelated children, the informality of home as opposed to the formality of school – but essentially the same principles of behavioural management are involved in both contexts. The parent or teacher is an agent involved in helping to shape the child's behaviour in certain directions and the direction in which the behaviour is shaped will depend to a large extent upon the types of behaviour which are being reinforced.

### Case study[1] (1)

Tony is a bright boy of seven. He is the youngest of three children. He has a brother aged 16 and a sister of 14. As the baby of the family Tony has always been somewhat indulged. He doesn't like it if he doesn't get his own way and recently he has developed a habit of becoming silent and unresponsive if something upsets him. The reaction of his parents has been to pay him a lot of attention when he begins to sulk in this way, treating him as if he was feeling unwell. They would ask him if he's feeling all right and offer him enticements of various sorts: 'Poor old Tony, are you all right?/Do you want to lie down?/Course you can have a go on John's guitar, can't he John?/Would you like a sweetie? Or a biscuit?' Unfortunately, by settling for an easy life (as they thought) and indulging Tony's whims when he was being awkward the parents were, in fact, reinforcing the very behaviour they were trying to avoid!

The cycle of behaviour was broken eventually by changing the consequences following Tony's sulks. Instead of letting him have his own way, or appeasing him with sweets or biscuits, the effect of which was essentially to reward the sulk and to increase the frequency of its occurrence, the family now adopted a different approach. They ignored him completely when he became sulky and transferred their special attention away from this unwanted behaviour to occasions when he was behaving well, i.e. they

---

1   The case studies are based on real individuals or situations but the names and some minor details have been changed in order to preserve anonymity.

concentrated on reinforcing his good rather than his sulky behaviour. After a few weeks, the effect of this new approach was that Tony's periods of good behaviour increased, his sulking decreased and relationships within the family became much more harmonious.

This tendency to reinforce unwanted behaviour patterns without realising it is a very common feature of parental and teacher behaviour, and one which explains a great many disciplinary problems at home and school. In most family environments, of course, the nature of the interaction between the parents and children is not analysed in this sort of way. Parents react spontaneously to their children's behaviour and *vice versa*, without thinking whether the consequences of their actions are likely to create more difficulties for them in the long run; and in most situations both children and parents survive the ordeal without too many disasters! In cases of difficult and repeated behaviour problems, however, it is useful to examine exactly what patterns of interaction lead to the emergence of the behaviour and what consequences usually follow its occurrence. This is sometimes called the ABC approach to behaviour management.

In the ABC approach, the *antecedents* of the behaviour are first examined (i.e. the events immediately preceding the occurrence of the problem behaviour); then the precise nature of the *behaviour* itself is pin-pointed (e.g. 'starting to cry when not given the same colour crayon as Mary' rather than just 'being naughty'); and finally the *consequences* of the behaviour are considered, particularly in terms of the actions engaged in by parents or teachers following the behaviour (e.g. whether they pay extra attention to the child, or ignore the behaviour). In Tony's case, the antecedents of one particular sulk involved Tony appearing uninvited in John's bedroom when John was trying to do his revision homework, with his school-books all around him on the bed. Tony started to strum John's guitar whereupon John told him to leave it alone. Tony then began to engage in his difficult behaviour, first stamping his feet and then sitting on the books on John's bed with his arms folded, eyes looking at the floor, in a silent sulk. Finally, the consequences were that the boys' mother, having heard the exchange from across the landing, came into John's bedroom. Seeing Tony sitting on the bed looking very doleful she went up to him and gave him a cuddle, saying 'Poor old Tony, 'Course you can have a go on John's guitar, can't he John?'

By examining the sequence of events in this sort of detail it becomes clear that Tony is actually being rewarded for his sulking and this is increasing the frequency of its occurrence. By adopting a revised and consistent family approach to the problem behaviour, it then becomes possible to find ways of changing the pattern of events to one which produces a more desirable behavioural response on the part of the difficult child. In this instance, for example, as already described, the new family policy was aimed at trying to change the nature of the consequences so that instead of rewarding Tony's sulk by giving him cuddles and sweets, they now ignored it and concentrated instead on rewarding his good behaviour.

As in schools, most families will find that it is useful to establish an agreed set of rules for certain situations (e.g. deciding what constitutes a late night out, and agreeing that the teenager will phone home if the time is likely to be significantly exceeded) but whether the rules are explicit or implicit one factor of over-riding importance in achieving a comfortable level of discipline is that the agreed rules should be applied consistently. The importance of consistent parental handling in helping to produce well-adjusted children is a very well-researched finding – erratic and inconsistent parental handling emerging as, for example, one of the most significant features in the backgrounds of young delinquents (Brooks 1985 p. 306). The existence of agreed rules, consistently applied within the framework of a loving home will provide a feeling of security for the child. Knowing the limits of expected behaviour is sometimes a frustrating experience but it can also offer a welcome degree of certainty in an uncertain world.

## Discipline in the school

As we have already seen, in examining children's behaviour it is important to consider the context in which the behaviour takes place. If we focus only on the child rather than the 'child in context' then we are likely to miss some important clues about the nature of the observed behaviour. For example, any head teacher will be able to point to children who behave like angels with one teacher but like devils with another. It is the same children reacting to a different set of circumstances; and the differences in the children's behaviour is a result of their responses to different teachers using different (or sometimes indifferent!) management techniques. As the Elton Report (Department of Education and Science (DES) 1989) on Discipline in Schools argued 'Group management skills are probably the single most important factor in achieving good standards of classroom behaviour'.

Quite often, as we have seen with Tony in the case study already described, it is the unintentional reinforcement of a child's 'bad' behaviour by the parent or teacher which acts as the 'trip wire' causing the behavioural problems to become even more recalcitrant. I have described this vicious circle elsewhere in this way:

> The stressed teacher...will inadvertently reinforce 'difficult' behaviour by paying undue attention to the petty misbehaviour of attention-seeking children rather than to their less frequent (but from a management point of view often more crucial) episodes of 'good' behaviour. This then leads

to an increase in the attention-seeking behaviour and to further teacher stress!' (Povey 1993)

The tendency for parents and teachers to label children as 'difficult' or 'disruptive' can also mitigate against the maintenance of good discipline since this practice tends to invite both the child and the parent or teacher to react in accordance with the stereotype. In other words, the parent or teacher comes to expect the pupil to behave in a certain way and, in an all too depressingly familiar scenario, the pupil invariably responds to the expectation! It is the same process which I have previously described in relation to the crude labelling of children as 'academic' or 'non-academic' at the 11+ stage of education and in which 'pupils tend to take on the stereotyped performance and behaviour of the class or school to which they have been allocated' (see Povey 1980, p.19). However, if teachers keep in mind (and get to know) the child as an individual rather than as a stereotype and attend to some basic guidelines in classroom management techniques such as those outlined, for example, in Wheldall, Merrett and Russell (1983), Fontana (1985), Bull and Solity (1987) and Varma (1993) then maintaining classroom discipline can become much less of a problem. In particular, emphasis needs to be placed on the following types of teaching skills:

- developing good individual relationships with the pupils both inside and outside the classroom, and being able to 'have a laugh' with the children

- preparing teaching materials carefully for each period so that the pupils are fully and meaningfully occupied

- using the voice effectively and ensuring that oral instructions are given clearly and precisely

- keeping alert to what is happening in all parts of the classroom, frequently 'scanning' the room even when occupied with individual pupils

- practising effective questioning and presentational techniques

- involving the children in worthwhile and challenging activities which are matched to the pupils' levels of understanding

- maintaining fairness and consistency in handling pupils' breaches of any agreed classroom rules

- making frequent use of positive reinforcement wherever possible both for good behaviour and good work and making sparing (but consistent) use of reprimands and sanctions.

Strong support for the value of such teaching skills as an aid to the maintenance of good classroom discipline is provided by the Elton Report. Drawing on their review of relevant research findings and examples of good practice in schools, the Report highlights the relevance of group management skills for teachers but opines that their importance has tended 'to be underestimated by teachers and their trainers' (DES 1989, p. 67). The Report also highlights the importance of teachers analysing their own classroom management performance and learning from such analyses. It is by modifying teaching approaches in the light of such self-critical appraisal (aided by discussions with experienced colleagues) that individual teachers can begin to make real improvements in their teaching techniques. Such improvements will help in the long term to reduce levels of teacher stress, improve teacher-pupil relationships generally and reduce the frequency of disciplinary problems. They will also help to ensure that the pupils are engaged in effective and enjoyable learning experiences.

An understanding and well-organized teacher using good group-management skills and working within the framework of a carefully thought out school disciplinary policy can work wonders even with the most recalcitrant of pupils, as can be seen by the experience of one multi-cultural primary school in London.

## Case studies (primary)

CASE STUDY (2)

This case study is based on the 'whole-school policy' developed at a large infant/junior school with over four hundred pupils, many of whom were bi-lingual. The policy is described in detail in Coulby and Coulby (1990).

The staff at the school wished to develop a whole-school discipline policy involving consultation at all stages with pupils and staff. In order to achieve this, each class initially discussed the idea of a set of rules which would support 'a happy safe school environment' and this was followed up by a meeting of the whole school at which the plan was further discussed. The pupils were encouraged to come forward with suggestions from their own classroom discussions and then a list of forty of these suggestions was displayed in a book which was available to all the pupils. After the pupils and staff had spent time discussing these ideas each class was asked to decide which three rules were, in their view, the most important rules from a list of 14 which had itself been reduced from the original 40, following discussion with the whole school at a special assembly. Four rules were finally selected for use in the school. These were:

1. We will be friendly and gentle with everyone and play safely together.

2.  We will be nice to each other about all the ways in which we are different.

3.  We will tell someone else as soon as we can if something is worrying us.

4.  We will listen to the adults who look after us and try to do what they ask straight away. (Coulby and Coulby 1990, p.48.)

The rules were widely displayed and communicated to parents and each class made a presentation in Assembly which was based on the operation of the rules. The essential key to the development of this successful policy was that the whole school, both staff and pupils, were involved in agreeing and establishing appropriate rules of behaviour. As the authors put it: 'A whole-school policy necessitates the development of a shared attitude towards the children, an acknowledgement of their equal rights and individuality. The point of the policy is to remove difficulties which might prevent any child reaching her/his highest possible potential. Its aim will be to skill children with alternative productive and appropriate behaviour.' (Coulby and Coulby 1990, p.48.)

CASE STUDY (3)

This case study, relating to the management of playground behaviour, is based on a project reported by White (1988). For a fuller discussion of approaches to discipline in the playground see Docking (1990) pp.92–5.

The primary school was in an educational priority area and great efforts were made to involve pupils, teachers, support staff and parents in evolving the playground policy. After numerous discussions a set of four rules was agreed. These were:

1.  We will always be kind and considerate to everybody in the playground.

2.  We will look after the playground and make sure that it is always a nice place to be in.

3.  We will share the playground space so that other games, besides football, can be played.

4.  Even if we are in the midst of something very exciting or important, we will stop and listen to any instructions an adult may give us. (White 1988, pp.197–8.)

In the cases of persistent offenders the parents were invited to come to the school so that the child's behaviour could be discussed with them. The project was time-consuming but rewarding, and, as Docking puts it 'the process of general participation itself seems to contribute to resolving the problems'. (1990, p.95)

## Behaviour modification

The teaching skills which are most likely to promote a good working atmosphere with a minimum of disciplinary problems within the classroom are essentially similar whether we are dealing with pupils in the primary or secondary school. The general principles have already been discussed, and they will be applicable within the context of any whole-school discipline policy which is based on the reinforcement of appropriate pupil behaviour, irrespective of the actual school rules selected.

However, in situations where the pupils' behaviour has become extremely difficult to manage it is sometimes worth considering the implementation of specific class management techniques which have been found to be effective in handling 'difficult' children. As an illustration of one such technique, I shall concentrate in the next case study on the description of a school setting in which a 'token economy' system has been used very successfully. The system is based on the principles of behaviour modification which also underpin the ABC approach described earlier. In simple terms, behaviour modification draws attention to the fact that behaviour which is reinforced tends to be repeated whereas behaviour which is unrewarded or penalised tends to be reduced (see Fontana 1985 Ch. 4; Harrop 1983; Wheldall *et al.* 1983). Thus behaviour-modification techniques attempt to 'shape' the behaviour of pupils by the use of appropriate reinforcements and penalties. Experiments in behaviour modification of this type are not uncommon in residential schools dealing with emotionally disturbed pupils (*see* e.g. Youell and McGinty 1984) but there is no reason why 'token economy' systems should not sometimes be tried in primary or secondary mainstream settings or at home, if the participating staff or parents find the system attractive for specific situations which have proved unresponsive to other measures. In the following case study the 'token economy' system was introduced in order to try to turn around a situation in which discipline had become extremely lax and both teachers and pupils were suffering from the effects of poor pupil behaviour.

### Case study (4) (secondary)

This study is based on a project reported by Fraser (1985).

The co-educational secondary school had been experiencing problems with band C pupils in the first and second years. These children were allocated to the C band because they required remedial support for their difficulties in language and mathematics. Many of these pupils 'had built up an antipathy and in some cases open hostility to school life'. The children tended to be noisy, disorganized, disruptive, forgetful and, in general, unmotivated and awkward to teach. After considerable discussion it was decided to introduce a 'token economy' system for these pupils for a trial period. The impetus to introduce such a system came from discussions between the teachers and the educational psychologist who had arranged a visit to a nearby residential special school for children with behavioural difficulties. In this special school a 'token economy' system had been operating with success for several years. The pupils had agreed with the teacher a few basic rules to which the class was expected to adhere, such as respecting each others' property and completing tasks which the teacher had set. During the week each pupil earned tokens with which they could 'buy' one of a selected range of personal-choice activities at the end of the week. Pupils could also lose points by breaking the rules, and they could incur agreed punishments when the number of lost points reached a certain level.

Enthused by the reports of the visit to the special school, the Head teacher arranged a staff meeting at which the educational psychologist and interested staff members put forward suggestions for introducing a 'token economy' system initially as a pilot scheme with one of the second year classes (2C). Then the proposals were discussed with the pupils and an agreed method of operating the system was worked out.

The staff wished to concentrate on improving the pupils' preparation for lessons and reducing the degree to which disruptive pupils interfered with other pupils' work. So it was agreed that there would be four basic classroom rules which emphasised that

1.　pupils must come to each lesson with a pen, pencil and ruler

2.　they must not disturb anybody else

3.　they must show respect to other people at all times

4.　they must complete set assignments to the best of their ability.

The selection of rules in a 'token economy' system is, of course, essentially determined by identifying the type of behaviour the school wishes to promote and marrying this to the type of behaviour which the teachers believe is reasonably manageable (and 'scorable') in the teaching context. For example, a more or less silent classroom may be a desirable and feasible objective in one situation but less appropriate in another. In this situation the staff and pupils agreed that the four rules seemed workable and appropriate.

The rules were clearly displayed in each classroom which 2C was using and during the lessons each member of the team of teachers involved completed a chart for each of the pupils taught. The pupils were given a grade of Good, Satisfactory or Poor depending upon their behaviour during the lesson. Each pupil started out with a G grade but when a pupil broke one of the rules he or she would be told that the rule had been broken and marked down on the sheet as an S. This would be done in a very cool, detached and matter-of-fact way without any suggestion of an implied threat. It was simply the teacher carrying out the agreed classroom rules. This detachment in implementing the rules is seen as a crucial element in the 'token economy' approach. Pupils who did not break any rule would gain a grade of Good at the end of the lesson, pupils who had broken a rule once would get a grade of Satisfactory, pupils breaking rules twice would get a Poor grade and pupils who continued to break the rules were marked down as an X grade and given 'time out'. This meant that they were sent to the Year Head (to be given what the participating staff describe as 'an icy reception') and then returned to their class for the beginning of the next lesson. Each child was given his or her grade at the end of each lesson, a new chart being completed afresh for each new lesson. Pupils who had gained a Good grade would be given positive reinforcement by being congratulated at the end of the lesson. Towards the end of the week the pupils' record charts were examined. Pupils whose charts had all Good grades (or 3 or fewer S grades with no P or X grades) were then given a free choice of activity during one afternoon. Care was taken to ensure that this did not appear as a type of punishment for the rest of the class – simply that the 'free choice' pupils had worked extremely well during the week.

For pupils who had a bad grade record, on the other hand, certain sanctions were employed. For example, if a child had been sent out during the week he or she would attend a detention for half an hour to make up for the time spent out of the lesson. Two detentions in any full 'grade period' (defined as half a term) resulted in the pupil being required to see the class teacher, Year Head and Deputy Head and being told that if he or she were given another detention then their parents would be approached. After three detentions the parents or guardians would be invited to discuss the child's behaviour.

The team of teachers involved with the 'token economy' system worked closely together and monitored the effects of the project carefully, making minor modifications to the system as they progressed. In general, it achieved its objectives of improving the working atmosphere of the classroom. Very few pupils forgot their equipment for lessons, their attitude to work improved as did the quantity and quality of work produced. In comparison with a control group of parallel pupils not using the system the pupils in the 'token economy' class also showed greater improvement in academic self-image and sociometric status (*see* Fraser 1985). Not all pupils liked the system. Some found it a bit condescending: 'I have not coped very well with this system so far. I think this is babies kind of thing. I agree about the equipment but the rest is just silly!' However, quite a number appreciated the improvement in working conditions: 'I think with our system we get our work done more quickly than we used to. The people that found it difficult to keep quiet are getting on with the system really well.' 'I think the system is great. It is the best thing which has happened to me in my whole school life. The new system has helped me to work faster now.' Following its adjudged success with 2C the system was extended to other classes in the following year.

## The problem of bullying

Bullying can be seen as 'the wilful, conscious desire to hurt, threaten or frighten someone' (Tattum and Herbert 1990, p.3). In a recent survey of 6758 primary and secondary aged pupils in Sheffield, it was found that 43 per cent reported being bullied in the year leading up to the survey. Contrary to the folk-lore that 'sticks and stones will break my bones but words will never hurt me' the research also suggests that children and adolescents seem to find indirect verbal bullying (especially 'having rumours spread about oneself') to be particularly distressing. Other sources of severe stress were 'being physically hurt, being called names, being deliberately left out or ignored and being threatened' (Sharp 1995, p.84).

The Elton Report suggests that teachers should 'be alert to signs of bullying and racial harassment; deal firmly with all such behaviour; and take action based on clear rules which are backed by appropriate sanctions and systems to protect and support victims' (DES 1989, p.103). Since that Report was published several projects have been set up to examine the problems of bullying, including the Sheffield project discussed earlier (*see* Sharp 1995; Sharp and Smith 1994). Some of the approaches to bullying have involved staff and pupil collaboration, along the lines of the discipline policies already described; and of particular interest are the schemes involving peer counselling and mediation. The 'mediation approach' has been growing in the UK in recent years both in schools and in the wider community.[2] It is described by Stacey (1996a) as 'a structured process in which a neutral third party assists voluntary participants to resolve their dispute... It allows the disputants to define the problem from

---

2   The 'umbrella' organisation co-ordinating mediation projects in the UK is Mediation UK, 82a Gloucester Road, Bishopston, Bristol BS7 8BN Tel: 0117 924 1234. The school mediation courses described in the case study on p.135 were organised by Hilary Stacey. She can be contacted at Catalyst, 5 Cambridge Road, Kings Heath, Birmingham B13 9UE Tel: 0121 4411222.

their point of view, identify and express their feelings and needs, hear the feelings and needs of the other person, acknowledge each other's point of view, create solutions, agree a course of action and evaluate progress at the end if necessary.'

*Case study (5)*

This is based on the scheme of peer mediation developed in Birmingham by Hilary Stacey (1996a,b)

A group of 14 primary and secondary schools in Saltley, Birmingham have recently committed themselves to using peer mediation in order 'to create a community-wide approach to reducing conflict and promoting positive relationships in their schools' (Stacey 1996b). Several of the staff at each school have been trained to supervise the mediation procedure in a series of two-day courses, and some of the teachers have also been released to write curriculum materials designed to teach the skills of mediation to their pupils. These skills have been identified as affirmation (the ability to recognise one's own and other people's strengths), co-operation, communication, listening and mediation. The training for mediation emphasises the 'whole school' approach and involves all pupils and staff 'reviewing their attitudes towards conflict and their behaviour in conflict situations from minor disputes to bullying and matters of classroom discipline... Children play co-operative games and learn to see everyone in their class as someone they should care about. They look at the things that they do that escalate and de-escalate conflict and learn mediation skills through role-play practice' (Stacey 1996a). The youngest pupils to be taught mediation skills in the UK so far have been eight-year-olds.

Although the scheme is in its infancy it has built on the success of previous work in other primary schools in Birmingham in which effective mediation has taken place in relation to name-calling and bullying, playground disputes (resulting in a fifty per cent reduction in the number of incidents being referred to the Head during lunchtimes) and disputes in library periods. Stacey (1996a) also reports that similar schemes in the USA have resulted in 'a 70 per cent decrease in suspensions for fighting' in one high school and 'a 47 per cent drop in aggressive behaviour' in another.

## Excluding pupils from school

Bullying, violence and other forms of disruptive pupil behaviour have created difficult problems for head teachers, and there has been a substantial increase in the number of children excluded from school during the 1990s (see Hayden

1994; Parsons 1994, 1996). Particular concern has also been expressed in these reports at the number of exclusions from primary schools.

### Case study (6)

The following case was reported in *The Times Educational Supplement* in November, 1994 (see Williams 1994):

Martin was seven when he was indefinitely excluded from his primary school for repeatedly stabbing another child with a compass. When his temper was roused, 'he would plunge the nearest object into the nearest person,' according to his head teacher. Although the boy was not 'consistently bad' his behaviour was unpredictable. 'That is where the danger lay,' says the head who runs a tough junior school in Kent. Other children were terrified of him. 'We had parents ringing up threatening to take their children away because of the fear factor.' Some acted on their fears – four children were withdrawn because of the disruption to their schooling. 'The local authority advised us to lock up our Stanley knives,' according to the head. 'But how can you assume that every potential weapon is safe and secure?'

Martin was referred to a behaviour guidance unit with plans for a gradual re-entry back into the school. But he never returned – over a three-year period his behaviour was never deemed to have improved enough.

Unfortunately Martin's case is not an isolated instance in Britain in the 1990s and the increase in young children's disruptive and often violent behaviour is a cause for concern, as too is the problem of leaving excluded children as 'debris outside the system' (Parsons *et al.* 1994, p.50). In an age when schools are increasingly being subjected to 'market forces', head teachers are increasingly unlikely to tolerate the presence of disruptive pupils within their schools. Such pupils will blacken the image of the 'product' and so make it difficult to sell to potential parental 'customers'. As Hayden (1994) puts it: 'The competition that has…been deliberately fostered between schools' (by the 1988 Education Reform Act and the 1993 Education Act) 'has not been developed with the needs of the 'less marketable' child in mind… In particular, formula funding and published league tables positively discourage schools from taking on and/or retaining children who contribute little to the performance indicators for a school.'

In a study of eleven children who had been excluded from primary schools Parsons *et al.* (1994) paint a picture of vulnerable (and often violent) children being excluded from school for long periods of time without adequate support or supervision. The average length of exclusion was 145 days, the equivalent of three-quarters of the school year; and the longest period of exclusion was two years for a child who was aged six when first permanently excluded.

Whilst teachers blame the parents, and the parents blame the teachers, the child roams the streets out of the control of a range of unco-ordinated 'authorities' – and few agencies are likely to act swiftly in this situation as can be seen by the case study below. Because of financial constraints 'short-staffed, under-resourced and over-loaded agencies' (such as the social and health services, social security and the police) 'are, in effect, having to ration their services' (Parsons *et al.* 1994, p.33).

*Case study (7)*

This is based on one of the 11 cases studied by Parsons *et al.* (1994).

The boy, who had been subjected to sexual abuse at home (as had his three brothers), was exhibiting severe behavioural and educational problems at school.

In January 1989, with his parents' consent, the boy was referred by the head teacher to the School Psychological Service for assessment of Special Educational Needs (with a view to statementing). The head teacher explained to the parents why the referral was being made, and they gave their consent to this course of action.

The educational psychologist had been swamped by referrals of cases of children suspected of being victims of sexual abuse and did not get round to following up the referral until December 1989. After the educational pyschologist's visit a variety of support was provided for the child and his family such as ancillary support in the classroom, assistance from the special needs teacher already within the school, psychiatric therapy at a clinic, support from Social Services.

In November 1990 the boy was excluded from school. This was made permanent and formal assessment was initiated. Unfortunately, through pressure of work, the educational psychologist did not manage to see the boy for assessment until February 1991 and when he did see him he used one of the tests which had already been carried out (without the psychologist's knowledge) at the Child Psychiatry Centre a few months earlier.

In May 1991 the educational psychologist completed his assessment (referred to as a pre-draft statement) with various suggestions about suitable educational provision. Several meetings involving professionals from different agencies were held with the child and his family. However, the approach to his problems was not co-ordinated and, in the view of Parsons *et al.* (1994, p.34): 'The response to the needs of child and family was inadequate.' They argue that it was clear in 1991 that this child would need to be statemented because of his special needs.

In July 1993 the pre-draft statement was still on file and it was not until December 1993 that the full statement was finally agreed; but, after nearly three years of exclusion, the child was still not in school!

So no one wants to know about the problems if they can avoid them; delay, 'cost-shunting' and procrastination are the order of the day. Finally, when the problem is eventually tackled the case has become much more expensive and the measures taken to deal with it are likely to be considerably less effective than they would have been if the child had been supported *within the school system*! Whatever actions are eventually taken, however, the problem of behaviourally-disordered children will not go away. Such children will continue to pose challenges to parents and teachers. As McManus argues, 'troublesome behaviour is as much a part of a teacher's job as it is of a parent's. Teaching is one of those professions which has a responsibility to respond to unco-operative persons in intelligent and considered ways' (McManus 1993, p.230). In other words, we should aim to reduce the degree of 'buck passing' which goes on in the system between agencies, and we should try to find ways of responding with a much more cooperative and coordinated approach to the problems of children with severe behaviour disorders. In studies based at Canterbury Christ Church College in Kent, Dr Carl Parsons is currently attempting to examine the effects of establishing co-ordinated, inter-agency support for children at risk of exclusion; and it is through monitoring such support systems, rather than by increasing the numbers of early exclusion orders, that we are likely to find the most effective ways of dealing with behaviourally disordered children.

## Conclusions

It is a trite comment, but nevertheless worth re-stating, that, in general, the best form of discipline is self-discipline; and one of the best ways in which to encourage children and adolescents to become self-disciplined is to allow them to enter into the responsibility of setting the ground rules for disciplined behaviour. As McManus argues: 'for some pupils, the new experience of being taken seriously improves their self-esteem and makes possible a change in their behaviour' (McManus 1993, p.231). But setting agreed rules of behaviour is only the beginning; it is then essential that these rules are consistently and fairly applied, whether this is within the home or at school. With a consistent and co-ordinated approach to the treatment of troublesome children, one which treats each individual with respect and has at its core the aim of getting to know the person behind the symptoms, it should be possible to improve disciplinary approaches and to reduce the number of children who are abandoned as 'debris outside the system'.

# References

Brooks, R. (1985) 'Delinquency among gifted children.' In J. Freeman (ed) *The Psychology of Gifted Children*. Chichester: John Wiley.

Bull, S.L. and Solity, J.E. (1987) *Classroom Management: Principles to Practice*. Beckenham: Croom Helm.

Coulby, J. and Coulby, D. (1990) 'Intervening in junior classrooms.' In J. Docking (ed) *Education and Alienation in the Junior School*. Basingstoke: The Falmer Press.

Department of Education and Science (DES) (1989) *Discipline in Schools*. Report of the Committee of Enquiry chaired by Lord Elton. London: HMSO.

Docking, J. (1990) *Managing Behaviour in the Primary School*. London: David Fulton Publishers.

Docking, J. (1993) 'The management of behaviour in primary schools.' In V. Varma (ed) *Management of Behaviour in Schools*. London: Longman.

Fontana, D. (1985) *Classroom Control: Understanding and Guiding Classroom Behaviour*. London: Methuen in association with The British Psychological Society.

Fraser, M. (1985) 'An examination of the effects of behaviour modification on sociometric status and academic self-image in a group of first year secondary school pupils.' Unpublished M.A. dissertation, University of Kent at Canterbury.

Harrop, A. (1983) *Behaviour Modification in the Classroom*. Sevenoaks: Hodder and Stoughton.

Hayden, C. (1994) 'Primary age children excluded from school: a multi agency focus for concern.' *Children and Society 8*, 3, 257–273.

McManus, M. (1993) 'Discipline in pupils excluded from school.' In V. Varma (ed) *Management of Behaviour in Schools*. London: Longman.

Parsons C. (1996) 'Permanent exclusions from schools in England in the 1990s: trends, causes and responses.' *Children and Society 10*, 177–186.

Parsons, C. with Benns, L., Hailes, J. and Howlett, K. (1994) *Excluding Primary School Children*. Family Policy Studies Centre, London, supported by Joseph Rowntree Foundation.

Povey, R. (1993) 'The psychological assessment of behavioural difficulties.' In V. Varma (ed) *Management of Behaviour in Schools*. London: Longman.

Povey, R.M. (ed) (1980) *Educating the Gifted Child*. London: Harper and Row.

Sharp, S. (1995) 'How much does bullying hurt? The effects of bullying on the personal well-being and educational progress of secondary aged students.' *Educational and Child Psychology (Selected Papers) 12*, 2, 81–88.

Sharp, S. and Smith, P.K. (eds) (1994) *How to Tackle Bullying in Your School: A Practical Handbook for Teachers*. London: Routledge.

Smith, R. (1985) *Freedom and Discipline*. London: George Allen and Unwin.

Stacey, H. (1996a) 'Mediation into schools does go! An outline of the mediation process and how it can be used to promote positive relationships and effective conflict resolution in schools.' *Pastoral Care in Education 14*, 2, 7–9.

Stacey, H. (1996b) 'Peer mediation: skills training for life.' *Primary Practice 3*, 10–14.

Tattum, D. and Herbert, G. (1990) *Bullying: A Positive Response*. Cardiff: South Glamorgan Institute of Higher Education.

Varma, V. (ed) (1993) *Management of Behaviour in Schools*. London: Longman.

Wheldall, K., Merrett, F.E. and Russell, H. (1983) *The Behavioural Approach to Teaching Package (BATPACK)*. Birmingham: Centre for Child Study, University of Birmingham.

White, P. (1988) 'The playground project: a democratic learning experience.' In H. Lauder and P. Brown (eds) *Education in Search of a Future.* Basingstoke: The Falmer Press.

Williams, E. (1994) 'When school can do no more.' *Times Educational Supplement,* 25 November.

Youell, S. and McGinty, J. (1984) 'The special group at Fairfield House.' *British Journal of Special Education 11,* 4, 13–15.

# CHAPTER 11

# Troubles of Young Offenders

*Robert Povey and Tim Emms*

Young offenders should be caned live on prime time television...just before the lottery draw! They should be treated toughly and seen to be treated toughly.

Home Secretary calls halt to 'golf course' prisons.

Detention no answer to youth crime – police chief.

Adventure holidays provide useful therapy for delinquents.

Tory Government to pilot 'boot camp' scheme for young offenders.

These headlines illustrate the type of media reports prevalent at the time we started writing this chapter. They represent the views of a range of people concerned, in one way or another, with the treatment of young offenders. At one extreme are what might be called the 'birching brigade': people who hold the view that the best way to deal with most criminals is to beat them or, more generally, to make them suffer for their crimes. As Elizabeth Peacock (Conservative MP and magistrate) put it in a speech in March 1995:

> We may not wish to cut off hands as seems to be common for thieves across the Arab world, but we could [seek] the reintroduction of the birch, [the introduction of] super prisons where prisoners are confined for 23 hours a day, no recreation, no socialising and no work...and campaign for the return of the death penalty.

These attitudes contrast sharply with the type of views expressed by people whom Edward Pearce (1994) contemptuously dismisses as 'the contemporary do-gooders' and 'compulsive understanders', people who look beyond punitive measures towards a better understanding of the causes of crime and of ways of rehabilitating the offender.

Much of the debate about the treatment of young offenders has taken place in the political arena where constructive debate has often been replaced by pontificating polemic. Strident calls for the re-introduction of the birch and for the incarceration of young offenders in secure units have contributed nothing to our understanding of the causes of criminal behaviour or to our evaluation of the effectiveness of different methods of rehabilitation. They simply aim to satisfy society's desire for punishment and revenge and ignore the evidence which suggests that regimes based on 'punitive' methods are less effective at preventing re-offending than those based mainly on educational and rehabilitative approaches to the young offender. We shall examine the evidence on this issue in the second part of the chapter. To begin with, however, we will consider some of the factors which lead to children becoming delinquents.

## Why do some young people become delinquent?

### Social factors

Theories about the roots of delinquency are many and varied but they revolve essentially around the twin influences of heredity and environment. There is a great deal of evidence to suggest, for example, that the child's environment exerts a strong influence on the likelihood of the development of antisocial and delinquent tendencies. Research studies have highlighted a number of predictors within the family backgrounds of young offenders. Social factors such as low family income, large family size and 'broken homes' have been shown to be related to a higher incidence of delinquency together with factors such as poor scholastic achievement. (See, for example, Glueck and Glueck 1950; West and Farrington 1973; West 1982). Tumim (1995) suggests that a 'hard core' of prisoners (around 80 per cent or so) have poor educational records and are underachievers (many being illiterate), and that around 40 per cent have been in care or have had 'difficult' home backgrounds. Similarly, there is a tendency for delinquents to have poor self-concepts (see Burns 1982, p.352) although, as we have argued elsewhere, delinquency can also sometimes be seen as a form of compensatory action adopted *in order to enhance self-esteem* (Emms, Povey and Clift 1986).

The fact that delinquency is usually defined in terms of those young people who are actually caught and convicted of a criminal offence rather than the total group of (apprehended and non-apprehended) offenders does, of course, create certain problems in interpreting data collected on delinquency. Thus it is quite possible that some of the youngsters who manage to escape detection (and hence by definition do not form part of the 'delinquent' sample) may be brighter, come from homes which are not 'broken' and find themselves somewhat better off than their convicted counterparts! This 'skewing' of the available statistics in the direction of unsuccessful offenders will clearly tend to distort our views about the characteristics of youngsters taking part in delin-quent activities; and there is some evidence, for example, that the relationship between 'broken homes' and engagement in delinquent activities is less strong amongst unconvicted offenders (Hennessy, Richard and Berk 1978). Never-theless, robust examination of the evidence does suggest that social factors *are* strongly implicated (in interaction with the other factors discussed later in the chapter) in the aetiology of delinquent behaviour (see, for example, Hollin 1993).

This conclusion is reinforced by the findings from the *Cambridge Study in Delinquent Development* (Farrington and West 1993; Farrington 1995) which identified six major theoretical constructs which are predictive of delinquent behaviour. As can be seen, at least half of these clearly come within the definition of 'social factors'. The six categories can be summarised as follows:

○ antisocial child behaviour, including troublesomeness in school, dishonesty and aggressiveness

○ hyperactivity and impulsive behaviour with poor attention span/concentration and a daring, restless demeanor

○ low intelligence and poor school attainment

○ family criminality, including convicted parents, delinquent older siblings and siblings with behaviour problems

○ family poverty, including low family income, large family size and poor housing

○ poor parental child-rearing behaviour, including inconsistent, harsh and authoritarian discipline, poor supervision, parental conflict and separation from parents.

These factors were the most important predictors at age 8–10 years of later delinquency (whether assessed by self-report or by actual convictions) amongst a group of 411 London males, mostly born in 1953, who have been followed through as part of a prospective longitudinal survey from the age of 8 to 32 years. (See Farrington 1995 for a review of key findings to date.) Out of the 411 males there were 24 chronic offenders who committed half of all the recorded offences for this sample. The most important risk factors for *chronic* offending were 'being seen as troublesome' (by teachers and peers) and as 'daring' (by parents and peers), having a parent who had been convicted of an offence and having a delinquent sibling. Confirmation of several of these factors also comes from a recent study of 92 persistent offenders in Kent (Weir 1995). The sample consisted of offenders between the ages of 12 and 17 who had been the subject of three or more police files in one year. Eighty per cent of offenders were regular truants and the same proportion had been excluded from school; 40 per cent were school bullies, 65 per cent had bad relations with their parents, 39 per cent had convicted parents, there had been alcohol and drug abuse amongst the offenders, and one third of the subjects had been on the Child Protection Service's 'at risk' register.

The link between crime rate and unemployment is another factor highlighted by data from the Cambridge study. The official crime rate for this group of subjects during periods of unemployment was roughly three times as great as it was when the subjects were employed (Farrington *et al.* 1986). The authors also emphasise that this increase in offence rate was confined to crimes involving financial gain (e.g. theft and burglary) whereas other offences such as violence and drug use did not increase during periods of unemployment. They conclude that the increase in crime rate is likely to be related in large measure to offenders' lack of money. Indeed the most common reason given by the boys themselves for delinquent activity is 'material gain' (Farrington 1993); but, since the next most frequently quoted reasons for committing offences are 'excitement, for enjoyment or to relieve boredom', it seems clear that these factors are also likely to play a strong contributory role in any increase in delinquent behaviour during periods of enforced leisure. This view is reinforced by self-reported (as opposed to official) offending figures which suggest that, in addition to financial gain, the search for excitement, usually in the company of other young people, is a potent motivating source for adolescent crime. For example, in an interview study of 74 persistent young offenders Hagell and Newburn (1994) found that one of the most commonly reported offences (after theft for material gain) was taking cars for 'joyriding'.

The effects of traumas during birth and early childhood are stressed by Raine, Brennan and Mednick (1994). In a longitudinal study of 4269 boys born in a Copenhagen hospital between 1959 and 1961 the researchers discovered a marked association between violent behaviour during the teenage years and earlier parental rejection and birth trauma. They found that the presence of birth complications such as breech births and forceps deliveries, coupled with parental rejection in the first year of life resulted in a predisposition to violent offending at the age of 18. Children who suffered only one of the early traumas were no more likely than average to develop violent behaviour patterns but the 4.5 per cent of children who were subjected to both were responsible for 18 per cent of the violent crime committed by the group. Professor Raine suggests that it may be that birth defects result in mild brain damage which in turn can lead to impaired intellectual ability, poor school achievement and a greater likelihood of unemployment, all factors which help to predispose adolescents towards criminal activities. On the basis of this evidence he also argues that better antenatal and perinatal health care, especially to mothers from poor socio-economic backgrounds, and follow-up parental support might help to reduce the incidence of violent teenage delinquents.

The antecedents of violent and aggressive teenage behaviour have also been examined by Farrington (1989) who concludes that such behaviour is most clearly predicted by the six broad factors mentioned earlier in our discussion of the *Cambridge Study in Delinquent Development:* antisocial behaviour, hyperactive and impulsive behaviour with poor attention span, school failure, family criminality, economic deprivation and poor child-rearing practices. The importance of family dynamics in the aetiology of delinquency is also emphasised in other studies of adolescent behaviour. For example, the effects of parental handling on teenage behaviour was examined in a sample of 90 Canadian male adolescents (65 of whom were young offenders) between the ages of 12 and 18 (see Truscott 1992). In this research it was found that the experience of child abuse in the form of *paternal* violence was strongly associated with the expression of violent behaviour on the part of the adolescents. Similarly, Loeber and Stouthamer-Loeber (1986) identified 'a harsh, rejecting style of parenting' as one of three broad features of problem families, the other two being large family size and parental disharmony. In a recent critical review of the influence of these factors, Hollin (1993, p.143) concludes that 'the parental style of discipline in "delinquent families" is typically lax, erratic, inconsistent, harsh and overly punitive'. He also concludes (p. 142) that the 'link between family size and delinquent behaviour holds true for studies using either official or self-reported measures of delinquency' and that 'the relationship between broken homes and delinquency has remained stable over time'. He notes, however, that it is not always clear exactly how such factors exert their influence on the development of criminal tendencies. With family size, for example, is it the tendencies for children in large families (defined by West and Farrington (1973) as four or more children) to be more socially disadvantaged, to receive less parental attention and to be less well supervised than children from smaller families which leads to a greater likelihood of the occurrence of delinquent behaviour? Or is it the greater likelihood within such families of having a delinquent sibling? The most probable explanation is that it is a combination of factors within the general notion of 'family size' which gives rise to the association with delinquency; but the 'contagion hypothesis' which suggests that delinquent behaviour 'rubs off', as it were, from one delinquent sibling to impressionable brothers or sisters (usually brothers) is certainly likely to be a significant feature in many cases of 'large family' delinquency, as in the case of Jason.

CASE STUDY[1] (1)

Jason was the youngest in a family of nine children and went to the same school for children with mild learning disabilities which was previously attended by two of his brothers. One of his older brothers was on probation for theft and another had been taken to court for an incident involving a dangerous weapon (a knife stolen from the grocers in which he worked). Jason had also been in trouble with the police in relation to taking a bicycle but was not charged with any offence. His father, a long-distance lorry driver was frequently away from home and somewhat remiss in providing 'housekeeping' funds for the family. When he was at home he was a very dominating figure, quick to react to cheeky or insolent behaviour by the use of abusive language and sometimes, though not generally, physical violence. Mother was more indulgent with the children but could also become very upset by events, and suffered badly with 'nerves'.

The mother confided to her GP about some small pilfering episodes at home, and the GP referred Jason to the Child Guidance Clinic. He was examined at the age of 12 by the educational psychologist who found him to be intellectually retarded and emotionally immature. He noted that Jason had very few close friends at school, tended to be antisocial and to engage in disruptive behaviour in class which he thought was probably an attention-seeking ploy. Despite his lack of friends at school he appeared to be greatly influenced by his brother, the one who had recently been taken to court. This brother was seen by Jason as something of a role model and Jason hung around with his brother's friends who encouraged him to engage in petty pilfering from local shops. Eager to please his brother and encouraged by all the attention his exploits engendered Jason took part in many of these small scale crimes.

When tested on the Wechsler Intelligence Scale for Children Jason's full scale IQ was in the mid sixties. He could manage easy arithmetical calculations and was capable of handling everyday monetary transactions in shops, but his reading ability was extremely limited. He was followed up from time to time at school by the Psychologist and by the Child Guidance psychiatric team which tried to offer support for the family.

The efforts of the school and support workers during Jason's teenage years seemed to have helped in keeping him from too much involvement with the police, although the 'contagion effect' with his brothers and their older mates continued to lead him into episodes of delinquent activities.

---

1   The case studies are based on the actual records of young offenders but, apart from the cases of Mary Bell, Jonathan Venables and Robert Thompson who have already been the subjects of published biographical studies (e.g. Sereny 1995), the names of the offenders and some minor details have been changed in order to preserve anonymity.

After leaving school he worked as an unskilled labourer in several jobs but his work record was unsatisfactory.

At the age of 19, however, without having shown any previous evidence of violence apart from one fracas at school a few years before, Jason suddenly became involved in a violent murder. Whilst on probation for theft he took a sharp kitchen knife which he claimed was for self-defence and wandered over to some local woods wearing his old hooded anorak. There he met a girl and ended up stabbing her to death. He pleaded guilty to manslaughter on grounds of diminished responsibility, was convicted and ordered to be detained in a prison hospital.

This case study illustrates many of the social factors which operate in the background of young offenders: the large family, financially impoverished, inconsistent discipline at home, family members involved in criminal activities (with two delinquent siblings), and peer group pressure from his brothers' friends who formed part of a delinquent sub-culture involving frequent truanting from school, pilfering, drug, alcohol and solvent abuse. It also illustrates the difficulty of predicting the likely occurrence of violent crime, and especially murder. Jason was not in general a 'violent' person in his actions. He was described by his sister as a 'very gentle' boy whom she often used as a babysitter. He was certainly an impressionable boy with very limited intellectual powers. He was also prone to engage in attention-seeking behaviour and his performance in the woods, like his disruptive behaviour in school could be seen as a 'daring' bid for attention. Or it could simply have been, as appears likely from the evidence at the trial, that the situation simply got out of hand and he panicked. Whatever the reason for his violent behaviour, it is difficult to see how this unexpected stabbing could have been anticipated in any precise way, or what preventive measures the probation officer currently in charge of his case could have taken in order to forestall this particular incident.

This difficulty in predicting the long-term future behaviour of youngsters identified at an early age as 'at risk' is highlighted by another study from the Cambridge research group (Farrington, Gallagher and Morley 1988). Fifty-six subjects identified as 'potential delinquents' at age 8–10 on the basis of such risk factors as low family income, large family size, convicted parents, low intelligence, and poor parental child-rearing behaviour, were followed up at the age of 32 years. The identification procedure worked well in the short term in the sense that three-quarters of this group had been convicted of criminal offences during adolescence and early adulthood. However, when studied at age thirty-two, half of the 56 subjects were leading what were described as 'successful lives', that is, they were adjudged to be showing satisfactory social adjustment. The researchers reported that the subjects 'were without convictions and other deviant behaviour, had good relationships with wives and children, and good accommodation and employment histories'. Their involvement with family commitments appeared to have induced a more responsible attitude towards offending. As far as the non-offenders in the sample were concerned they differed from the offenders in having less contact with other boys and an absence of convicted fathers and delinquent siblings. Despite remaining unconvicted and generally being well-behaved, however, they were not necessarily leading the most 'successful' lives when assessed on the criterion of social adjustment.

Thus the evidence suggests that it is possible to make *broad* predictions about the likelihood of groups of 'vulnerable' youngsters engaging in delinquent activities during adolescence and early adulthood, but, as Jason's case illustrates, it is far from easy to predict the *specific* behavioural outcomes in individual cases. Jason's history also illustrates three other characteristics which are associated with delinquent behaviour: low intelligence, poor scholastic achievement and the tendency for boys to outnumber girls in any delinquent group by estimated ratios varying between 3 to 1, and 10 to 1 (Commins 1971). These characteristics, together with the whole range of personality variables which distinguish one individual from another, are often discussed under the general heading of 'individual differences'.

### Individual differences and the role of hereditary factors

When looking at the role of individual differences as a factor in the aetiology of delinquency we are moving into the 'heredity' end of the heredity/environment spectrum. This is not to say that all individual differences in cognitive functioning and personality are genetically determined but that genetics has a strong role to play in interaction with environmental factors in influencing the behaviour of young people during their formative years. It seems likely that some children inherit a propensity to develop certain behavioural characteristics such as aggressiveness or impulsivity just as they can inherit a tendency to develop certain forms of intellectual impairment. But the way in which such propensities develop is determined by their interaction with the environment.

Much of the recent interest in the influence of genetic factors in the aetiology of criminal behaviour comes from studies by Brunner *et al.* (1993a; 1993b). Working in the Department of Human Genetics at the University Hospital in Nijmegen, Holland, Brunner and his colleagues studied a Dutch family over four generations in which the males tended to be intellectually retarded and to exhibit impulsive aggressive behaviour resulting in a high incidence of crimes such as arson and attempted rape. They found that the affected males had a genetic abnormality of the X chromosome which, they argued, could be one of the factors influencing their behaviour patterns. Brunner's work has also been influential in another case which has focused attention on hereditary factors in the aetiology of criminal behaviour. This is the case in the USA of Stephen (Tony) Mobley, a convicted armed robber and murderer. During his trial the defence counsel appealed against the imposition of the death sentence on the grounds that Stephen Mobley's behaviour was caused by his genetic inheritance which had predisposed him to a life of violence. His family tree revealed a catalogue of violence and antisocial behaviour going back at least four generations and the lawyers argued that Mobley should be allowed to undergo genetic testing and that this evidence should be accepted in court as a valid defence. The Georgia Supreme Court ruled in March 1995 that these tests were not permissible in Mobley's case, but the defence arguments highlight the way in which genetic factors are now increasingly being acknowledged as important players in the aetiology of criminal behaviour.

The work of Raine, Venables and Williams (1990) has also provided interesting indications of the way in which genetic predisposition to criminality may find its expression in certain patterns of brain dysfunction. Raine and his co-workers have found, for example, that criminal behaviour in adulthood is related to certain neuro-psychological phenomena, in particular to under-arousal of both the central and autonomic nervous systems during adolescence. One hundred and one male schoolchildren between 14 and 16 years of age were tested on psychophysiological measures in 1978–79. Ten years later, 17 out of the original 101 subjects were found to have criminal records and the psychophysiological data obtained in their teens showed that these young men had significantly lower arousal levels on EEG, cardiovascular and electrodermal measures. The argument advanced by Raine is that messages in the brain (particular those activating the pre-frontal cortex) which enable an individual to focus attention and to regulate or control emotional behaviour are *underpowered* in these individuals; and, paradoxically, the tendency is for such people to compensate for this under-arousal by seeking out an excessive degree of stimulation and excitement which can sometimes lead to criminal activity. As Adrian Raine put it in a recent Channel 4 television programme *A Mind to Crime: The Dangerous Few* (screened in the UK on 3rd October 1995): 'kids with low arousal seek out stimulation to increase their arousal level back to normal' and he surmised that for some adolescents using a gun, committing a burglary or beating someone up might be their way of pepping up their arousal levels. A number of such delinquents have been diagnosed as having what is known as an attention deficit disorder (ADD), often with the addition of hyperactive tendencies, and there is an increasing body of research evidence to suggest that ADD, which has the familiar low arousal patterns described by Raine, may be implicated in the aetiology of some forms of criminal behaviour (Moffitt 1990;

Forehand *et al.* 1991; Satterfield *et al.* 1994).[2] There is also some indication that it may be possible to reduce a few of the behaviour problems arising from under-arousal patterns by the use of appropriate and carefully monitored stimulant medication (Barkley, DuPaul and McMurray 1991; Rapport *et al.* 1994; Barrickman *et al.* 1995; Spencer *et al.* 1995). However, as Hinshaw (1992) remarks, 'medication alone rarely provides clinically sufficient benefits' and it seems likely, as he goes on to argue, that the most effective results will be achieved by linking medication to social, psychological and educational interventions with the children, their families and teachers (see also Satterfield, Cantwell and Satterfield 1979).

Such evidence supports the argument that genetic factors can lead to certain patterns of brain dysfunction which may have an important part to play in the determination of some forms of criminal behaviour. But it would be quite inappropriate to conclude from this that there is a 'gene for crime'. It is highly likely that some people are predisposed to develop certain behaviours which could lead to criminal activities (see Brennan and Mednick 1993; Moore and Jessel 1995) but whether and to what extent such a predisposition does actually lead to crime will depend upon the interaction of these heredity factors with the environmental influences to which the person is exposed.

## The effects of screen violence on children and adolescents

On 12 February 1993 two-year-old James Bulger was lured away from a shopping precinct to a place a couple of miles away near a railway line where he was brutally murdered. The killing was carried out by two ten-year-old boys, Robert Thompson and Jon Venables. They battered Jamie to death with bricks and an iron bar causing forty-two separate injuries. Both boys were known to social workers and exhibited many of the features which are commonly found in the background of young offenders. For example, they were low achievers scholastically, troublesome at school, persistent truants and from 'broken homes'. But one aspect of the case gave rise to particular discussion. This was the suggestion by the trial judge that the boys' behaviour may have been affected by watching violent videos such as *Child's Play 3* in the home. Sereny (1995, p.316) argues that 'Mr Justice Morland had a very clear purpose when he brought up the point of violent videos in the home: he wanted to remind us that children are malleable and highly subject to influences, particularly now from films. Stable children – and adults – exposed to violent films, run the danger of becoming emotionally desensitized by a surfeit of such visual

---

2   A closely related syndrome called Conduct Disorder (CD) also appears to exhibit a strong pattern
    of cross-generational transmission (Frick 1994) and is even more clearly predictive of delinquent
    behaviour than ADD (Lie 1992).

experiences, but they are unlikely to be harmed by them. Unstable children, however, from chaotic backgrounds, are extremely susceptible to their mesmerizing effect.'

Research evidence about the effects on children of watching violent films or television programmes is somewhat equivocal. For example, in a study involving 1565 adolescent boys in London, Belson (1978) demonstrated that those subjects exposed to most violence on television committed a significantly higher proportion of violent acts, whereas Gauntlett (1995) concludes from his review of some of the relevant literature that the case for screen violence having a direct effect on violent behaviour is not proven. Indeed, this whole research area is fraught with experimental and ethical difficulties which make it hard to conduct meaningful studies of the effects of screen violence on children; and, in addition, many of the existing studies were carried out before television programmes and videos depicting scenes of extreme brutality (the 'video nasties') became freely accessible to young children. Nevertheless, Sims and Gray (1993) point to 'more than 1000 papers, linking heavy exposure to media violence with subsequent aggressive behaviour' and Bailey (1993), in a review of 40 adolescent murderers and 200 young sex offenders concluded that repeated viewing of violent and pornographic videos appeared to be one of the background factors affecting the behaviour of some of these young offenders.

What seems clear from the debate following the James Bulger murder trial is that some young children have a much greater access to video nasties, and watch them on a more regular basis, than had been previously assumed to be the case. It also seems likely that the content of much mainstream, prime-time television has become more violent in recent years. A recent survey of television programmes by the Broadcasting Standards Council, for example, revealed that 52 per cent of terrestrial television programmes and 73 per cent of programmes transmitted by satellite channels contained scenes of violence (Broadcasting Standards Council 1994; Culf 1994). Although there is some evidence of slightly more rigorous self-regulation by the television companies since this survey was undertaken (Gunter and Harrison 1995), the apparent preoccupation with violence both in news programmes and drama productions on television and in videos has undoubtedly led to a more dangerous 'home entertainment' climate for children whose viewing habits are poorly supervised. As Newson (1994, pp.273–4) argues:

> There must be special concern when children (or adults for that matter) are repeatedly exposed to images of vicious cruelty in the context of *entertainment and amusement* [and] there continues to be a need for systematic research in order to keep pace with both the growth of violence in children and the growth of violent visual material available.

Whilst the exact relationship between exposure to screen violence and the expression of violent behaviour in children and adolescents is still unclear, there can be no doubt that repeated exposure to screen violence is likely to have a desensitising effect on the viewer and that 'watching specific acts of violence on the media has resulted in mimicry by children and adolescents of behaviour that they would otherwise, literally, have found unimaginable' (Sims and Gray 1993). Thus the available evidence strongly suggests that watching violent films or videos should be taken seriously as one of the factors which may influence the behaviour of a proportion of violent young offenders. We would, therefore, agree with Newson's (1994) plea for more responsible parental supervision of children's viewing habits perhaps involving where appropriate a 'V' (or 'violence') chip incorporated into the television receiver as an aid to the regulation of children's viewing. We also strongly endorse her view that we need a much greater degree of research funding to examine the impact of video violence on the behaviour of children and adolescents.

## How should young offenders be treated?

> There was no talking except on Saturday and Sunday afternoons. On weekdays there was an hour's PT, marching around, like a boot camp. You had three books a week which you couldn't change, and punishment for changing a book was bread and water. It was emotional deprivation to break the will down.

This is the description of treatment in a Borstal institution in the mid-twentieth century by Bruce Reynolds, one of the Great Train Robbers, as reported in a recent article in *The Guardian* (Campbell 1995). Reynolds' experiences form the basis of his book *The Autobiography of a Thief* (1995) in which he maintains that this type of hard-line approach to young offenders often simply results in the emergence of fitter and wilier delinquents, with a greater repertoire of 'criminal' skills and an even greater determination than ever to become career criminals! This view from the 'inside' receives some support from the evidence from recidivism studies. According to figures quoted by the Howard League and other penal reform organisations (*The Observer* 1994) the re-offending rate for young offenders placed in secure units is 85 per cent, whereas the rate for similar offenders dealt with within community schemes is much lower (55 per cent). As John Mortimer QC, President of the Howard League, put it in the context of a comment on the 1994 Conservative government's proposals to build more secure units for young delinquents:

> If millions of pounds of taxpayers' money is available to deal with teenagers who commit crimes, it would be more effective to invest in local services to keep children in school, support families, provide active

recreation, and other successful crime prevention measures. Penal institutions for children are schools of crime. (Mortimer *et al.* 1994)

The evidence that custodial training schemes, as compared with rehabilitative 'hostels', tend to lead to greater re-offending rates is also supported by comparison of individual institutions. For example, according to recent 'Key facts and figures about juvenile crime' (*The Observer* 1994) 'Lisnevin, a school in Northern Ireland which runs custodial training schemes for persistent offenders aged 12 to 15, has a reconviction rate of 85 per cent within two years of release', whereas one of the homes criticised for using individual rehabilitation techniques involving overland travel expeditions (Bryn Melyn, in North Wales) 'puts its re-offending rate at 20 per cent'.

The aim of treating young offenders more as individuals than numbers and seeking to increase the opportunities for developing personal relationships between staff and offenders is also supported by the former H.M. Chief Inspector of Prisons, Sir Stephen Tumim. In an Open Lecture at the University of Kent (Tumim 1995) he argued that in treating young offenders we should aim for a secure hostel atmosphere rather than a custodial prison climate. This view is reinforced by his successor as Chief Inspector of Prisons, Sir David Ramsbotham who advocates the setting up of separate establishments for juvenile and young offenders in order to eradicate the prevailing culture of bullying and violence in many young offenders' institutions (see *The Guardian*, 1997).

In general, we would support the view that it is better to try to deal with the young offender within a community setting wherever this is feasible, making effective use of a well-staffed and well-qualified Probation Service. At the moment many probation officers feel that their pleas for a more 'rehabilitative' approach fall on deaf ears:

> The refusal to listen has now brought virtually the whole of the criminal justice system to a point where consensus between ministers and those who carry out the Home Office's work has all but disappeared and many feel that progress is made despite, and not because of, government action... But now comes the saddest fact of all. An unnecessary increase in incarceration will only create more victims of crime as recidivism goes untackled; ill-advised measures like the withdrawal of pre-sentence reports and the building of secure training centres will do nothing constructive and will cost the taxpayer more; and the closure of bail hostels and the enforced reduction of cautioning will mean that more of our young people irretrievably enter a criminal class rather than being given the opportunity to find an exit before lasting damage is done. (Honeyball 1994)

There have been some interesting attempts to find ways of providing non-custodial treatment for young offenders such as the Community Support Scheme adopted in Hampshire (Field 1992). This project targeted young offenders who were likely to receive custodial sentences (mainly relating to burglary) and had no appropriate adult support in the community. The scheme, which operates on a voluntary basis, aims to provide a supportive intervention programme with pre-service training for the caregivers and involvement of the natural parents and other significant people in the youngster's lives. Another recent initiative in Kent points the way to the possibility of more collaborative approaches between the Police and Social Services (Weir 1995). The Intensive Supervision and Support Programme (ISSP) has been developed in which an individual package of help is provided for each persistent offender. A key aspect of this programme is education. At present, children excluded from school are only required by law to have three hours of tuition per week. The ISSP scheme intends to increase the education input for such children and to prioritise the return of excluded young people back into a school setting. Police involvement is also seen as crucial in this exercise of 'tough care'. For example, whereas at present children under supervision orders are only required by law to be seen once a week, those on ISSP will be seen at least two or three times weekly by social workers, and almost as frequently by the police in their supervisory capacity.

Constructive intervention of this sort, whether within or outside a custodial setting, is at the heart of any approach which attempts to modify the damaging life experiences which most young offenders have experienced. Indeed, as Bullock et al. (1990) make clear, even in secure units it is the 'background problems of entrants (e.g. poor social skills, low educational achievements, lack of motivation, shattered self-confidence)' which are the primary areas of damage which need addressing and for which the young offenders' families are unlikely to be able to offer any great degree of support.

This points to the crucial need for early intervention to counteract some of the detrimental effects which environmental disadvantages can bestow on 'vulnerable' children. For example, improved health facilities for children of pre-school age would help to reduce some of the casualties to which Raine and his research team (Raine, Brennan and Mednick 1994) have drawn our attention. There is also encouraging evidence that early intervention programmes with parents and Infant School teachers can be very effective in reducing aggressive tendencies in children (see, for example, Hawkins, Von Cleve and Catalano 1991; Hawkins et al. 1992). In this study both teachers and parents of first grade children (aged six) were trained to pay particular attention to the positive aspects of behaviour management, rewarding the children's participation in 'socially desirable behaviour' wherever possible rather than resorting primarily to punishment for non-desirable behaviour. The parents' programme, emphasising the need for positive reinforcement, was called 'Catch them being good'! By the fifth grade, children in the experimental group were less likely to have become delinquent than those in the control group. As Farrington (1990) argues, apart from pre-school intellectual enrichment programmes it seems likely that 'the most hopeful methods of preventing offending (are) behavioural parent training'.

CASE STUDY (2)

Roger was born into a large family in relatively poor financial circumstances. He had a poor record at school where he was constantly in trouble; his teachers told him he was thick and treated him as a 'no-hoper'. Not surprisingly, his level of self-esteem was extremely low and he abandoned any real efforts at schoolwork in favour of trying to gain approval from a group of delinquent peers. He began to engage in a number of daring exploits in order to impress his new mates and ended up, after 'tanking up on ale', in someone's house at the foot of the owner's bed with a sawn-off shotgun, demanding money. He was apprehended and ended up in a residential unit for young offenders.

In the unit his lack of self-confidence was very evident. He made little or no eye contact with the other inmates or the staff and considered that there was no point in him doing any 'education'. 'My teachers told me I'm thick. So it's no use trying to teach me anything. I won't understand.' Nevertheless he volunteered for a maths class and after six months his teacher put him in for a RSA Basic Numeracy exam. The teacher told him he didn't have to take the exam if he really didn't want to, but he added 'I think you can do it'. With this vote of confidence from his teacher Roger agreed to 'give it a go' and he emerged with an 'A' grade!

The effects of one teacher's belief in Roger's capabilities, Roger's own hard work and his success in one small 'basic numeracy' examination were remarkable. He developed a much greater belief in himself and his capabilities and actually asked if he could work for further examinations. These he subsequently passed with good grades.

After leaving the unit he found employment in a printing works, found a new set of mates and appears to have abandoned the delinquent sub-culture to date.

## Treatment for addiction

It is clear that many young offenders who find themselves 'inside' are suffering from health problems of various kinds (Bailey 1993), particularly problems of mental health (Kendall et al. 1992). According to Bailey the population of young offenders in residential accommodation population 'shows a much higher level of psychiatric disorder and gross neurological and behavioural disturbance than such a population 20 years ago...[and] there has been an increase in the suicide rate among young prisoners.' Amongst the most prevalent forms of ill health within groups of young offenders are addictions to alcohol, drugs, solvents and gambling, and these are areas in which people working with young offenders require an increasing level of expertise.

The relationship between excessive alcohol consumption and delinquent behaviour is well established (see Cookson 1992) and a number of successful 'alcohol education' programmes have been developed for young offenders with alcohol problems (see, for example, Baldwin *et al.* 1991). In particular, it has been shown that behavioural self-control training can effectively encourage moderate drinking and that this can be achieved through a variety of approaches such as the use of self-help manuals, developing peer interventions, and using simulated bar settings (McMurran 1991). The relationship between addictive behaviour patterns and delinquency also exists for other substances apart from alcohol (Cookson 1994) and for gambling (Huff and Collinson 1987), the drug abusers or gamblers frequently engaging in criminal activity in order to finance their habits. Hence rehabilitative programmes for drug abuse and gambling, along the lines of those already described for alcohol abuse, represent prime target areas for the funding of research programmes which aim to improve the treatment of young offenders.

## Conclusions

We have tried to show that the aetiology of delinquency is multi-factorial. Individuals inherit potentialities of certain kinds – for example, they tend towards aggressive or impulsive behaviour or they suffer from some type of minor neurological dysfunction – but the extent to which such potentialities lead to delinquent or other forms of 'deviant' behaviour will be determined by the environmental circumstances with which the person comes into contact. Where inherited predispositions are overlaid with disadvantaged environmental circumstances – such as an impoverished home background where other members of the family have criminal records; having violent, abusing parents; being subjected to inconsistent discipline at home; being labelled at school as 'thickies' and 'troublemakers'; failing to find employment after leaving school – then delinquent behaviour patterns are likely to emerge. But none of these factors, on its own, can be seen as the 'cause' of the delinquency. They are factors which, taken together, tend to act as breeding grounds for delinquent behaviour.

As far as the treatment of delinquency is concerned we would side with those who argue that the most effective approach is to tackle those environmental disadvantages which beset potential delinquents and which are susceptible to modification. So we must try to ensure, for example, that children (and their parents) have the most effective health facilities and family support services available to them in the early years of a child's life in order to reduce the number of children who begin life with the disadvantage of early childhood traumas of various kinds. Similarly, it becomes crucial that we help parents and teachers to find the most effective approaches to the management of children's behaviour and ways of providing the most appropriate curricular experiences for the less intellectually able pupils (Parsons 1993). By such means we may be able to prevent at least some vulnerable children from becoming complete 'no-hopers' irrevocably programmed to slip out of the educational process and into the delinquent sub-culture waiting for them outside the school gates.

With troublesome adolescents who have already become young offenders we would again place education at the centre of our approach to treatment. Educational interventions, both within the community and in penal institutions, should be seen as the essential elements in treating the young offender since education can be so influential in helping to develop life skills which in turn affect the individual's level of self-esteem and potential for finding some form of useful employment. Not all educational interventions will turn out to be as rewarding or influential as those in Roger's case study but education (from pre- to post-school settings) is undoubtedly one of the most powerful tools we have at our disposal in preventing the emergence of new generations of young offenders.

## References

Bailey, S. (1993) 'Health in young persons' establishments: treating the damaged and preventing harm.' *Criminal Behaviour and Mental Health 3*, 4, 349–367.

Baldwin, S., Heather, N., Lawson, A. and Ward, M. (1991) 'Effectiveness of pre-release alcohol education courses for young offenders in a penal institution.' *Behavioural Psychotherapy 19*, 4, 321–331.

Barkley, R.A., DuPaul, G.J. and McMurray, M.B. (1991) 'Attention deficit disorder with and without hyperactivity: clinical response to three dose levels of methylphenidate.' *Pediatrics 87*, 4, 519–531.

Barrickman, L.L., Perry, P.J., Allen, A.J., Kuperman, S., Arndt, S.V., Herrmann, K.J. and Schumacher, E. (1995) 'Bupropion versus methylphenidate in the treatment of attention-deficit hyperactivity disorder.' *Journal of the American Academy of Child and Adolescent Psychiatry 34*, 5, 649–57.

Belson, W. (1978) *Television Violence and the Adolescent Boy*. Farnborough: Saxon House.

Brennan, P.A. and Mednick, S.A. (1993) 'Genetic perspectives on crime.' *Acta Psychiatrica Scandinavica 87*, (Suppl 370), 19–26.

Broadcasting Standards Council (1994) *BSC Monitoring Report II: 1993*. London: BSC.

Brunner, H.G., Nelen, M., Breakefield, X.O. and Ropers, H.H. (1993a) 'Abnormal behavior associated with a point mutation in the structural gene for monoamine oxidase A.' *Science 262*, 5133, 578–580.

Brunner, H.G., Nelen M.R., van Zandvoort, P., Abeling N.G., van Gennip A.H., Wolters,E.C., Kuiper, M.A., Ropers, H.H. and van Oost, B.A. (1993b) 'X-linked borderline mental retardation with prominent behavioral disturbance: phenotype, genetic localization, and evidence for disturbed monoamine metabolism.' *American Journal of Human Genetics 52*, 6, 1032–9.

Bullock, R., Hosie, K., Little, M. and Millham, S. (1990) 'Secure accommodation for very difficult adolescents: some recent research findings.' *Journal of Adolescence 13*, 3, 205–216.

Burns, R.B. (1982) *Self-concept Development and Education*. London: Holt, Rinehart and Winston.

Campbell, D. (1995) 'One of your very uncommon criminals.' *The Guardian*, 1st April.

Commins, N. (1971) *The Essence of Delinquency*. Cambridge: Cambridge Aids to Learning (Publishing) Ltd.

Cookson, H.M. (1992) 'Alcohol use and offence type in young offenders.' *British Journal of Criminology 32*, 3, 352–360.

Cookson, H. (1994) 'Personality variables associated with alcohol use in young offenders.' *Personality and Individual Differences 16*, 1.

Culf, A. (1994) 'TV standards.' *The Guardian*, 29 January.

Emms, T.W., Povey, R.M. and Clift, S.M. (1986) 'The self-concepts of black and white delinquents.' *British Journal of Criminology 26*, 4, 385–393.

Farrington, D.P. (1989) 'Early predictors of adolescent aggression and adult violence.' *Violence and Victims 4*, 2, 79–100.

Farrington, D.P. (1990) 'Implications of criminal career research for the prevention of offending.' *Journal of Adolescence 13*, 2, 93–113.

Farrington, D.P. (1993) 'Motivations for conduct disorder and delinquency.' *Development and Psychopathology 5*, 225–241.

Farrington, D.P. (1995) 'The twelfth Jack Tizard memorial lecture. The development of offending and antisocial behaviour from childhood: key findings from the Cambridge Study in Delinquent Development.' *Journal of Child Psychology and Psychiatry 36*, 6, 929–964.

Farrington, D.P., Gallagher, B., Morely, L., St. Ledger, R.J. and West, D.J. (1986) 'Unemployment, school leaving and crime.' *British Journal of Criminology 26*, 4, 335–356.

Farrington, D.P., Gallagher, B. and Morley, L. (1988) 'Are there any successful men from criminogenic backgrounds?' *Psychiatry 51*, 2, 116–130.

Farrington, D.P. and West, D.J. (1993) 'Criminal, penal and life histories of chronic offenders: risk and protective factors and early identification.' *Criminal Behaviour and Mental Health 3*, 4, 492–523.

Field, S. (1992) 'Young Offender Community Support Scheme – Hampshire, England.' *Community Alternatives International Journal of Family Care 4*, 2, 77–96.

Forehand, R.L., Wierson, M., Frame, C. and Kempton, T. (1991) 'Juvenile delinquency entry and persistence: do attention problems contribute to conduct problems?' *Journal of Behaviour Therapy and Experimental Psychiatry 22*, 4, 261–164.

Frick, P.J. (1994) 'Family dysfunction and the disruptive behavior disorders: a review of recent empirical findings.' *Advances in Clinical Child Psychology 16*, 203–226.

Gauntlett, D. (1995) *Moving Experiences: Understanding Television's Influences and Effects*. Academic Research Monographs, No. 13. London: J. Libbey.

Glueck, S. and Glueck, E.T. (1950) *Unravelling Juvenile Delinquency*. New York: Commonwealth Fund.

*The Guardian* (1997) 'Young offenders forced to fight off institution bullies to survive.' 11th March.

Gunter, B. and Harrison, J. (1995) *Violence on Television in the United Kingdom. A Content Analysis.* Unpublished research report, Department of Journalism Studies, University of Sheffield.

Hagell, A. and Newburn, T. (1994) *Young Offenders and the Media: Viewing Habits and Preferences.* London: Policy Studies Institute.

Hawkins, J.D., Von Cleve, E. and Catalano, R.F. (1991) 'Reducing early childhood aggression: results of a primary prevention programme.' *Journal of the American Academy of Child and Adolescent Psychiatry 30*, 208–217.

Hawkins, J.D., Catalano, R.F., Morrison, D.M., O'Donnell, J., Abbott, R.D. and Day, L.E. (1992) 'The Seattle social development project: effects of the first four years on protective factors and problem behaviours.' In J. McCord and R. Tremblay (eds) *Preventing Antisocial Behaviour.* New York: Guilford.

Hennessey, M., Richard, P.J. and Berk, R.A. (1978) 'Broken homes and middle-class delinquency: a reassessment.' *Criminology 15*, 505–528.

Hinshaw, S.P. (1992) 'Academic underachievement, attention deficits, and aggression: comorbidity and implications for intervention.' *Journal of Consulting and Clinical Psychology 60*, 6, 893–903.

Hollin, C.R. (1993) 'The lack of proper social relationships in childhood failure.' In V. Varma (ed) *How and Why Children Fail.* London: Jessica Kingsley Publishers.

Honeyball, M. (1994) Letter: 'Policies that lead young people along the road to crime.' *The Guardian*, 7 July.

Huff, G. and Collinson, F. (1987) 'Young offenders, gambling and video game playing.' *British Journal of Criminology 27*, 4, 401–410.

Kendall, K., Andre, G., Pease, K. and Boulton, A. (1992) 'Health histories of juvenile offenders and a matched control.' *Criminal Behaviour and Mental Health 2*, 3, 269–286.

Lie, N. (1992) 'Follow-ups of children with attention deficit hyperactivity disorder (ADHD): review of literature.' *Acta Psychiatrica Scandinavica 85*, (Suppl 368), 1–40.

Loeber, R. and Stouthamer-Loeber, M. (1986) 'Family factors as correlates and predictors of juvenile conduct: problems and delinquency.' In M. Tonry and N. Morris (eds) *Crime and Justice: An Annual Review of Research Vol 7.* Chicago: University Press.

McMurran, M. (1991) 'Young offenders and alcohol-related crime: what interventions will address the issues?' *Journal of Adolescence 14*, 3, 245–253.

Moffitt, T.E. (1990) 'Juvenile delinquency and attention deficit disorder: boys' developmental trajectories from age 3 to age 15.' *Child Development 61*, 3, 893–910.

Moore, A. and Jessel, D. (1995) *A Mind to Crime.* London: Michael Joseph.

Mortimer, J., Hardy, R., Harvey-Jones, J., Pannone, R. and Seabrook, R. (1994) Letter: 'Scars of the schools of crime.' *The Guardian*, 12 May.

Newson, E. (1994) 'Video violence and the protection of children.' *The Psychologist 7*, 6, 272–274.

*The Observer* (1994) 'Key facts and figures about juvenile crime.' 24 July.

Parsons, C. (1993) 'Inappropriate curricula, teaching methods and underfunctioning.' In V. Varma (ed) *How and Why Children Fail.* London: Jessica Kingsley Publishers.

Pearce, E. (1994) 'Bad guide for do-gooders.' *The Guardian*, 23 August.

Raine, A., Venables, P.H. and Williams, M. (1990) 'Relationships between central and autonomic measures of arousal at age 15 years and criminality at age 24 years.' *Archives of General Psychiatry 47*, 11, 1003–1007.

Raine, A., Brennan, P. and Mednick, S.A. (1994) 'Birth complications combined with early maternal rejection at age 1 year predispose to violent crime at age 18 years.' *Archives of General Psychiatry 51*, 12, 984–8.

Rapport, M.D., Denney, C., DuPaul, G.J. and Gardner, M.J. (1994) 'Attention deficit disorder and methylphenidate: normalization rates, clinical effectiveness, and response prediction in 76 children.' *Journal of the American Academy of Child and Adolescent Psychiatry 33*, 6, 882–893.

Reynolds, B. (1995) *The Autobiography of a Thief.* London: Bantam.

Satterfield, J. H., Cantwell, D.P. and Satterfield, B.T. (1979) 'Multimodality treatment: a one-year follow-up of 84 hyperactive boys.' *Archives of General Psychiatry 36*, 9, 965–974.

Satterfield, J., Swanson, J., Schell, A. and Lee, F. (1994) 'Prediction of antisocial behavior in attention-deficit hyperactivity disorder boys from aggression/defiance scores.' *Journal of the American Academy of Child and Adolescent Psychiatry 33*, 2, 185–90.

Sereny, G. (1995) *The Case of Mary Bell: A Portrait of a Child who Murdered.* London: Pimlico.

Sims, A.C.P. and Gray, P. (1993) *The Media, Violence and Vulnerable Viewers.* Document presented to Broadcasting Group, House of Lords.

Spencer, T., Wilens, T., Biederman, J., Faraone, S.V., Ablon, J.S. and Lapey, K. (1995) 'A double-blind, crossover comparison of methylphenidate and placebo in adults with childhood-onset attention-deficit hyperactivity disorder.' *Archives of General Psychiatry 52*, 6, 434–43.

Truscott, D. (1992) 'Intergenerational transmission of violent behavior in adolescent males.' *Aggressive Behavior 18*, 5, 327–335.

Tumim, S. (1995) 'Custody and community: policy for prisons in the 1990s.' Open Lecture, University of Kent at Canterbury, 24 February.

Weir, A. (1995) 'No future for crime.' *The Guardian*, 27 June.

West, D.J. and Farrington, D. (1973) *Who Becomes Delinquent?* London: Heinemann.

West, D.J. (1982) *Delinquency: Its Roots, Careers and Prospects.* London: Heinemann.

# CHAPTER 12

# Overview

*Maurice Chazan*

The contributors to this volume have discussed the troubles of children and adolescents from varying perspectives and have illustrated the many forms that these troubles can take. They have demonstrated that it is not easy to define and describe children's troubles (henceforth in this chapter, the term 'children' will include 'adolescents' unless otherwise indicated). In Chapter 2, for example, Helen Barrett and David Jones explain that even commonly used terms such as 'anger' mean such a wide range of different things to different people that there is surprisingly little agreement over the formulation of a precise definition. There has been much debate, too, over whether jealousy can be distinguished from envy (see Helen Barrett, Chapter 3).

The contributors have also shown how children react to their difficulties in different ways. Some children keep their troubles to themselves and cope with them, more or less, without causing any disturbance to anyone else, while others bottle their troubles up, but perhaps take refuge in withdrawal from aspects of life or in physical or mental illness. As Francis Dale (Chapter 4) asserts, the primary aim of withdrawal, which is a form of defence mechanism, is the avoidance of certain situations. Margaret Wright (Chapter 8) also views a depressive illness as offering a shell or protection from adversity, or an escape from a lifestyle that produces intolerable suffering.

Some children and adolescents openly publicise to those around them that they are troubled by being troublesome to others, through challenging authority at home and/or at school, failing to maintain positive relationships, bullying siblings or classmates, or becoming delinquent. Some are so overwhelmed by their personal turmoil that they are unable to pay attention to school work, as Howard Roberts (Chapter 9) shows, or resort to alcohol or drugs as a kind of sedative.

This overview will not attempt to summarise the content of all the previous chapters, but rather will focus on selected emphases in the book, under the following headings:

1. Causal explanations of the troubles of children and adolescents.

2. The importance of the close family unit.

3. The effects of a negative self-image.

4. Approaches to preventing or dealing with children's troubles.

5. Future research and developments.

## Causal explanations of the troubles of children and adolescents

All the writers in this book have acknowledged that the troubles of children and adolescents are rarely attributable to a single factor. Instead, combinations of factors are involved which have a unique impact on each individual. David Fontana (Chapter 7) has, for example, comprehensively discussed various causal explanations of troubles occurring in adolescence in terms of the psychoanalytic model, with its emphasis on early relationships between child and parent; the sociological model, stressing the importance of the social context in which events take place; the biological model, which underlines the effect of physical and physiological changes on development; the cognitive model, which suggests that a questioning mind and an idealistic stance may lead to impatient and intolerant behaviour; and the identity model, which highlights the crucial part played by an individual's self-image (see below for a further discussion of self-image). Fontana points out the strengths and weaknesses of each model and attempts to integrate them through the focal model, which sees the concerns emphasised by the other models as providing points of focus at different stages of development.

K. Eia Asen, in Chapter 1, while highlighting the key role of the family in most people's lives (see below for an elaboration of this point), acknowledges the part played by the school and the child's peers in the manifestations of troubled behaviour. Helen Barrett and David Jones (Chapter 2) and Helen Barrett (Chapter 3) highlight the influence of cultural values and expectations in the expression of feelings such as anger or jealousy as well as the effect of gender differences, but also see dispositional variables (such as temperament) and child-rearing practices as possible factors in causing disturbed feelings and behaviour in childhood and adolescence.

In his chapters on aggression (Chapter 5) and sexuality (Chapter 6), Francis Dale, while placing much stress on psychodynamic explanations giving prominence to the effects of problems of development in the early years, recognises that children's troubles are in part due to the erosion of extended family and community support for children. Dale also refers to the familial and cultural vacuum in which many children are brought up in, and the absence of moral values and traditions to guide them in the formation of responsible attitudes.

Howard Roberts (Chapter 9) and Robert Povey (Chapter 10) pay special attention to children's troubles related to school. Howard Roberts stresses that academic failure often occurs in association with mental health problems, and that the school environment may be of particular importance in conduct disorders. Sometimes, as stated above, the child is so troubled by personal worries and anxieties that he/she is unable to concentrate on school tasks; sometimes it is the case that failure to cope with the challenges set in school leads to difficulties in general adjustment. Robert Povey illustrates how erratic and inconsistent parental practices as well as faulty management in the classroom may be the antecedents of undesirable behaviour or serve to reinforce it.

In Chapter 11, Robert Povey and Tim Emms cite evidence for the strong, though not exclusive, influence of social factors in the development of delinquent tendencies. These factors include poverty and poor housing, defective parental child-rearing practices and family criminality. However, Povey and Emms, as do the other contributors, emphasise that the effects of environmental factors will vary in the case of each individual. It is important to take account of individual differences, partly determined genetically, in considering the causation of troubles in childhood and adolescence, although preventative measures and treatment strategies will tend to focus on environmental variables.

## The importance of the close family unit

In each chapter, whatever its main concern, the importance of the close family unit in the causation, prevention and management of children's troubles is highlighted. Because of the intimate and emotionally charged nature of family life, it is not surprising that there is plenty of potential for troubled relationships in each family, as K. Eia Asen states in Chapter 1. However, the family also has much potential for preventing troubles in children, and for helping to deal with them when they occur. Helen Barrett and David Jones (Chapter 2) present evidence to support the relationship between parental socialisation practices and children's ability to express negative emotions such as anger in socially acceptable ways. Jealousy may be almost inevitable on the birth of a sibling, but the manner in which parents deal with this event is likely to have a considerable influence on the feelings of a displaced child, as Helen Barrett suggests in Chapter 3. Barrett also points out that when children feel excluded, the person best suited to help them is the one they feel excluded by, and professional support must take this into account.

Francis Dale, writing from a psychodynamic viewpoint in Chapters 4, 5 and 6, puts a strong emphasis on the need, in therapy, to deal with unresolved conflicts and family relationships, particularly between mother and child, going back to the early years of life. David Fontana (Chapter 7), while recognising that insight into the problems of adolescence requires an understanding of a wide range of possible social factors, concludes that it is the micro-world of the family that provides the most important social context, rather than the macro-world of society at large, and that wise parenting remains of more consequence than any other single social variable.

The other authors reinforce the crucial nature of the close family unit. In Chapter 8, Margaret Wright asserts that parents can assist greatly in detecting the early signs of depression in their children, as well as in family therapy aiming to improve relationships at home. Howard Roberts (Chapter 9), while focusing on the links between psychiatric problems and a child's scholastic difficulties, emphasises that these links should not be considered in isolation from environmental factors such as the child's family. In Chapter 10, Robert Povey underlines the importance of consistent parental handling in helping to avoid maladaptive behaviour in their children; and, as mentioned above, Povey and Emms in Chapter 11 point to a number of factors related to the material and emotional aspects of family life which may lead to juvenile delinquency.

## The effects of a negative self-image

This book cogently testifies to the vital role played by a positive self-image in the development and maintenance of a relatively trouble-free childhood and adolescence. K. Eia Asen (Chapter 1) asserts that children who feel undervalued tend to seek to gain attention by clownish behaviour or to acquire a reputation for being tough. As Asen states, it is particularly those children who have no friendships who try to gain dubious popularity by carving out such identities for themselves. This point is also made by Howard Roberts (Chapter 9) and Margaret Wright (Chapter 8). Roberts shows that children who feel rejected by their peers and who consider that they are regarded by others with hostility frequently present conduct disorders and have a poor self-image in respect of their performance at school, where they often underachieve. Both Wright and Roberts highlight the loss of self-esteem and the holding of negative ideas about the self as a key characteristic of depression in childhood and adolescence. Poor self-concepts, perhaps related to a disadvantaged home background, a lack of success at school or rejection by most peers may lead to a youth seeking compensation through membership of a delinquent gang, where a sense of status may be experienced, as Povey and Emms (Chapter 11) assert.

In Chapter 3, Helen Barrett shows how jealousy presents a challenge to a child's sense of self in relation to important others, and may cause emotional damage through the child's feelings of betrayal: the jealous child perceives him/herself to be deprived of respect, love and admiration previously regarded as his or hers by right. In Chapter 7, Fontana underlines the need for an integrated sense of self during adolescence; failure to achieve the search for identity that is a prominent feature of this phase of development leaves the individual confused about his/her role in life. For further discussions of negative self-concept, see Beck and Freeman (1990) and Segal and Blatt (1993).

## Approaches to preventing or dealing with children's troubles

Everyone experiences troubles at some time or another, and children and adolescents cannot be wholly protected from such experiences. Many children, especially as they mature, will be able to cope with their troubles largely from their own resources. However, a considerable number will need some help, from their family, school or the support services, in order to maintain balance and order in their lives. If this fact is generally recognised, and if support for children is readily available at an early stage whenever necessary, then the adverse effects of children's troubles will be minimised. In the past, troubled or troublesome children have been too easily labelled in a negative way, and help has often been provided as a last resort, if at all. Much still remains to be done, but many families and schools are now more aware of the contribution they can make in pre-empting and managing troubles in childhood and adolescence.

This book suggests a number of ways in which families and schools can facilitate the prevention and treatment of maladaptive behaviour. The role of the close family unit in providing security and affection, consistent handling and encouragement as a basis for healthy development has already been mentioned in this overview. The family can give timely support to a child experiencing trouble by showing a sensitive understanding of the child's needs at the time, by being prepared to listen, and by a willingness to co-operate with the school and therapeutic agencies, should these be involved. As K. Eia Asen (Chapter 1) states, the parents' capacity to reflect on the thoughts, feelings and wishes of the child is crucial for the development of a positive parent–child relationship; the help of parents and other family members should always be sought to assist the child in trouble (see Hornby 1995 and Naomi Dale 1995 for discussions of ways of working with families of children with special needs).

The school is a powerful agency through which children's troubles can be minimised or managed. Schools need to be aware of the relationship between scholastic failure and mental health problems underlined by Howard Roberts in Chapter 9. They need to pay careful attention to learning difficulties if the adverse emotional consequences of such difficulties are to be avoided. Robert Povey (Chapter 10) highlights the relevance of group management skills for promoting the all-round development of individuals and for avoiding conflict and disruption in the classroom (see also Wragg 1993). Well-planned and agreed school policies ('whole school' policies) involve a consideration of what is to be done with those pupils who need special help, for whatever reason; strategies to prevent and deal with bullying; and a readiness to consult pupils, parents and the support services (see McManus 1995). The existence of a counselling service within schools can enable pupils to communicate their troubles to an understanding person instead of bottling them up (see McGuiness 1995). With appropriate guidance and assistance, for example from an educational psychologist, schools may be able to set up behaviour modification programmes of the kind illustrated by Povey in Chapter 10 (see also Wheldall and Merrett 1984).

Social skills training can also be helpful in avoiding troubles arising from, for instance, an inability to communicate effectively or a lack of competence in making or sustaining positive relationships with others. It is encouraging that many schools now assume responsibility, in collaboration with parents, for ensuring that children are able to cope with social relationships and with many of the problems that arise in the course of social interaction in daily life. Such schools regard social skills training as a part of the curriculum for all pupils, as well as setting up special projects such as training in 'peer mediation' outlined by Povey in Chapter 10 (see also Fontana 1990; Frederickson and Simms 1990; Roffey, Tarrant and Majors 1994; Nelson 1996).

Schools and institutions of further and higher education can also make a contribution to the treatment of young offenders in a community setting, as Povey and Emms show in Chapter 11. Education is often seen as a central aspect of programmes of rehabilitation, since many young offenders have a background of unsatisfactory experiences of the education system and need to be encouraged to adopt a more positive view of what education can offer them. Educational interventions can be very influential in raising self-esteem and increasing potential for employment.

The work of the psychiatrist in helping troubled children and their families is discussed in Chapters 1, 8 and 9 (see Chesson and Chisholm 1995 for an appraisal of the work of child psychiatric units) and Francis Dale gives examples of the ways in which psychotherapy in the psychoanalytic tradition can directly help a disturbed child or adolescent (Chapters 5, 6 and 7). Psychotherapy may be provided on an individual or group basis (see Dwivedi 1993 for a discussion of group work with children and adolescents) and through verbal interaction or play (see Cattanach 1994). Helen Barrett and David Jones (Chapter 2) give illustrations of intervention programmes based on cognitive behaviour therapy, rational emotive therapy and narrative therapy, all of which approaches aim to help a child to develop a greater awareness and understanding of emotional reactions (see Harris 1989).

## Future research and developments

In recent years, knowledge about the causes of children's troubles has greatly increased and current work is adding to the understanding of emotions such as anger and jealousy. Greater insight has been gained, too, into depression and anxiety states during childhood and adolescence (see Craig and Dobson 1995). The need now is to focus on how to prevent, minimise and intervene effectively in children's troubles. Current challenges include child abuse (Waterhouse 1996) and addiction to alcohol and drugs (see Silbereisen, Robins and Rutter 1995). A satisfactory answer has still not been found to preventing and dealing with juvenile delinquency. Further, as Fontana states in Chapter 7, the speed of technological change and the continuing decline of traditional values and moral codes are the two factors most likely to exacerbate problems.

In spite of many reports and initiatives, the level of co-operation between the many agencies dealing with troubled children still leaves much to be desired, and, as Povey (Chapter 10) stresses, a much more co-ordinated approach is needed. The *Code of Practice on the Identification and Assessment of Special Educational Needs* (DFE 1994) stresses that effective action on behalf of children with special needs will often depend upon close co-operation between schools, local education authorities, the health services and the social services departments of local authorities.

Research and experiment have suggested a wide variety of strategies that can be used to help children with troubles, and this book has given examples of many of these approaches. Far more evaluations of these strategies are needed, not only in an academic context but also through accounts of clinical practice as well as of carefully monitored school-based projects. Particularly in the educational system, practitioners are often too busy or too reluctant to publicise the interesting and valuable work which they undertake and need to be given incentives to make such work more generally known.

While many families cope reasonably successfully in spite of having to endure unsatisfactory basic living conditions, some of the troubles of children and adolescents stem from social disadvantage, including poverty and poor housing (see Chazan *et al.* 1977; Pilling 1990). Appropriate governmental action aimed at reducing material hardship, therefore, is likely to make a significant contribution to improving the general adjustment of a considerable number of children. Further, the provision of greater educational opportunities and the raising of educational standards, particularly in disadvantaged areas, will help the development and motivation of many young people who at present see little purpose in their lives (Barber 1995). However, no panaceas exist for the troubles of children and adolescents. As David Fontana (Chapter 7) emphasises, there is a need to avoid over-generalisations and to strive for a greater understanding of individual differences in reactions to problems and to the strategies used to solve them.

# References

Barber, M. (ed) (1995) *Raising Educational Standards in the Inner Cities: Practical Initiatives in Action.* London: Cassell.

Beck, A.T. and Freeman, A. (1990) *Cognitive Therapy of Personality Disorders.* New York: Guilford Press.

Cattanach, A. (1994) *Play Therapy: Where the Sky Meets the Underworld.* London: Jessica Kingsley Publishers.

Chazan, M., Cox, T., Jackson, S. and Laing, A.F. (1977) *Studies of Infant School Children, Vol. 2: Deprivation and Development.* Oxford: Basil Blackwell (for the Schools Council).

Chesson, R. and Chisholm, D. (1995) *Child Psychiatric Units: At the Crossroads.* London: Jessica Kingsley Publishers.

Craig, K.D. and Dobson, K.S. (eds) (1995) *Anxiety and Depression in Adults and Children.* Thousand Oaks, CA: Sage.

Dale, N. (1995) *Working with Families of Children with Special Needs.* London: Routledge.

Department for Education (1994) *Code of Practice on the Identification and Assessment of Special Educational Needs.* London: Central Office of Information.

Dwivedi, K.N. (1993) *Group Work with Children and Adolescents.* London: Jessica Kingsley Publishers.

Fontana, D. (1990) *Social Skills at Work.* London: British Psychological Society and Routledge.

Frederickson, N. and Simms, J. (1990) 'Teaching social skills to children: towards an integrated approach.' *Educational and Child Psychology* 7, 1, 5–17.

Harris, P. (1989) *Children and Emotion: The Development of Psychological Understanding.* Oxford: Basil Blackwell.

Hornby, G. (1995) *Working with Parents of Children with Special Needs.* London: Cassell.

McGuiness, J. (1995) *Counselling in Schools: New Perspectives.* London: Cassell.

McManus, M. (1995) *Troublesome Behaviour in the Classroom: Meeting Individual Needs,* (2nd edition). London: Routledge.

Nelson, V. (1996) 'Making an impact: social skills groups for secondary pupils.' *Educational Psychology in Practice* 12, 2, 107–111.

Pilling, D. (1990) *Escape from Disadvantage.* London: Falmer Press.

Roffey, S., Tarrant, T. and Majors, K. (1994) *Young Friends.* London: Cassell.

Segal, Z.V. and Blatt, S.J. (1993) *The Self in Emotional Distress: Cognitive and Psychodynamic Perspectives.* New York: Guilford Press.

Silbereisen, R.K., Robins, L. and Rutter, M. (1995) 'Secular trends in substance use: concepts and data on the impact of social change on alcohol and drug abuse.' In M. Rutter and D.J. Smith (eds) *Psychosocial Disorders in Young People: Time Trends and Their Causes.* Chichester: Wiley.

Waterhouse, L. (ed) (1996) *Child Abuse and Child Abusers.* London: Jessica Kingsley Publishers.

Wheldall, K. and Merrett, F. (1984) *Positive Teaching: The Behavioural Approach.* London: Allen and Unwin.

Wragg, E.C. (1993) *Classroom Management.* London: Routledge.

# The Contributors

**Ved P. Varma** was formerly an educational psychologist with the Institute of Education, University of London, the Tavistock Clinic, and for the London Boroughs of Richmond and Brent. He has edited or co-edited more than 35 books in education, psychology, psychiatry, psychotherapy and social work.

**K. Eia Asen** is a Consultant Child Psychologist at the Marlborough Family Service and Consultant Psychotherapist at the Maudsley Hospital, London.

**Helen Barrett** is Research Fellow of the Department of Psychology, Birkbeck College, University of London, and Senior Lecturer in Psychology at Thames Valley University.

**Maurice Chazan** is Emeritus Professor of Education at the University of Wales, Swansea.

**Francis Dale** is a Consultant Child and Adolescent Psychotherapist, Torquay.

**Tim Emms** is a Psychologist and was formerly Lecturer in Education at a Youth Custody Centre.

**David Fontana** holds posts as Professor in the Universities of Minho and of Algarve, Portugal, and is Distinguished Visiting Fellow in the University of Wales, Cardiff UK.

**David Jones** is a Senior Lecturer in Psychology, Birkbeck College, University of London.

**Robert Povey** is an Educational Psychologist and was formerly Principal Lecturer in Education at Canterbury Christ Church College.

**Howard Roberts** is a Consultant Child and Adolescent Psychiatrist, Lambeth Healthcare NHS Trust.

**Valerie Sinason** is a Consultant Child Psychotherapist at the Tavistock Clinic and a Consultant research Psychotherapist at St. George's Hospital Medical School.

**Margaret Wright** is a Consultant Child Psychiatrist in Buckinghamshire.

# Subject Index

ABC approach 126
'abnormality' definition 4–5
academic failure *see*
    learning problems
'accidents' and aggression
    80–1
addiction treatment 155–6
ADHD (attention deficit
    hyperactivity disorder)
    118–19
adolescence 96–107, 162,
    164, 165
    aggression in 72–4
    biological model 99–1
    cognitive model 102
    focal model 104–5
    identity model 103–4
    psychoanalytical model
        96–7
    sociological model 97–9
agency co-ordination
    136–8
aggressiveness 63–81; 161
    anger compared 16
    communication of 74–5
    contexts for 68–74
    and depression 109
    reasons for 63–8
    strategies for managing
        75–81
Alan, withdrawal case 46–7
alcohol and delinquency
    156
ambivalence, adolescent 97
'anal character' 88
anal stage 82, 88–9
anger 15–29, 161, 163
    cultural differences 16–18
    defining 15–16, 18–19
    in infancy 20

management techniques
    26–7
role of emotion 21–2
socialisation 24–6
temperament 22–4
'anger with oneself' 19
antidepressants 111
anxiety disorder 120–2
arousal levels, and
    delinquency 149–50
attachment 3–4
    and aggression 67–8
    and depression 112
    and temperament 23–4
    and withdrawal 60–1
attention deficit
    hyperactivity disorder
    (ADHD) 118–19
autism 47–8, 51
autonomy development 101
avoidant disorder 121

'battle for the breast' 85–6
befriending networks 41
behaviour modification
    techniques 131–4
behavioural role of
    emotions 21
'benign splits' 52–3, 79–80
Bible jealousy examples 30
biological model of
    adolescence 99–101,
    162
Birmingham peer
    mediation project 135
birth problems, and
    delinquency 144
body image problems 100
boundaries, personal 53
breast
    'battle' for 85–6
    'greediness' 87
    'loss' of 63–4
    as self 64, 83–4, 85
bullying 13, 134

Cambridge Study in
    Delinquent
    Development 143, 144,
    147
checking questions 11, 12
chronic offending 143
clarifying inquiries 11, 12
CCNES (Coping with
    Children's Negative
    Emotions Scale) 24–5
cognitive models of
    adolescence 102, 162
communication
    of aggression 74–5
    with withdrawn children
        53–4
community support 92–3,
    98
    of offenders 153–4
'compliant self' 49
conduct disorder 116–18,
    150
constitutional withdrawal
    45
containment 3, 65, 76
coping strategies, parental
    24–5
Coping with Children's
    Negative Emotions
    Scale (CCNES) 24–5
counselling service 166
covert aggression 74, 80–1
cultural differences
    anger 16–17, 162
    jealousy 39, 162

defence systems 40, 44–5
delinquency *see* offenders
depression 108–13,
    119–20, 161, 164
    diagnosis 109–10
    incidence 109
    prognosis 112
    treatment 110–12
developmental psychology
    approach to jealousy
    34–6
'devouring breast' concept
    87

170

# Author Index